GALVESTON COOKBOOK RECIPES

Nutrient-Dense Diets to Help You Achieve Your Health Goals

Dr. Veronica J. Reynoso

Table of contents

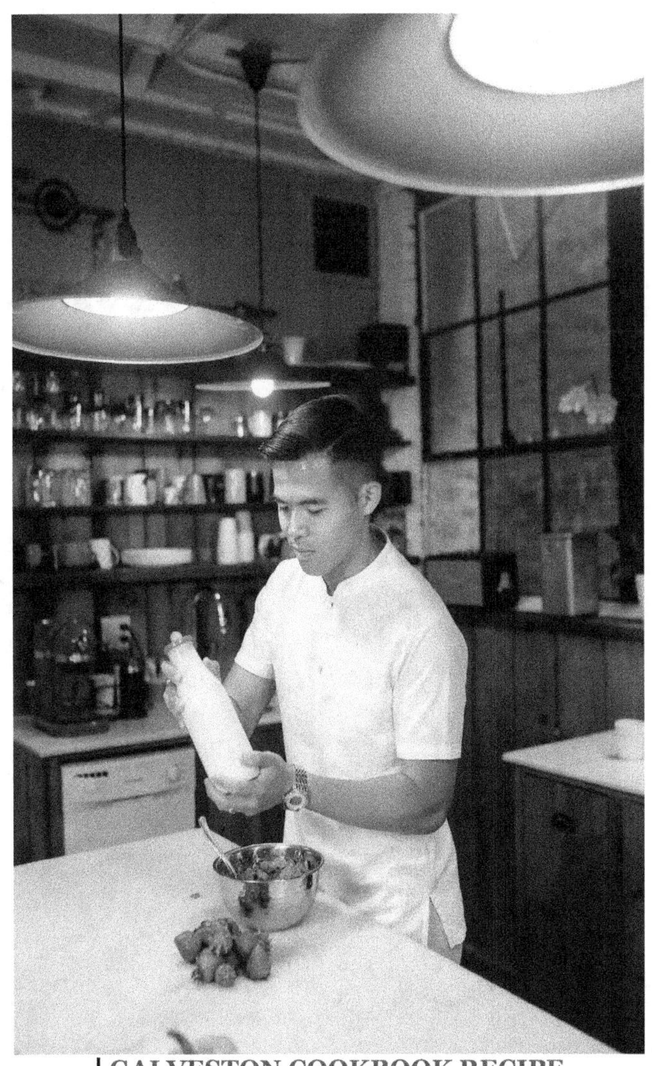

GALVESTON COOKBOOK RECIPE

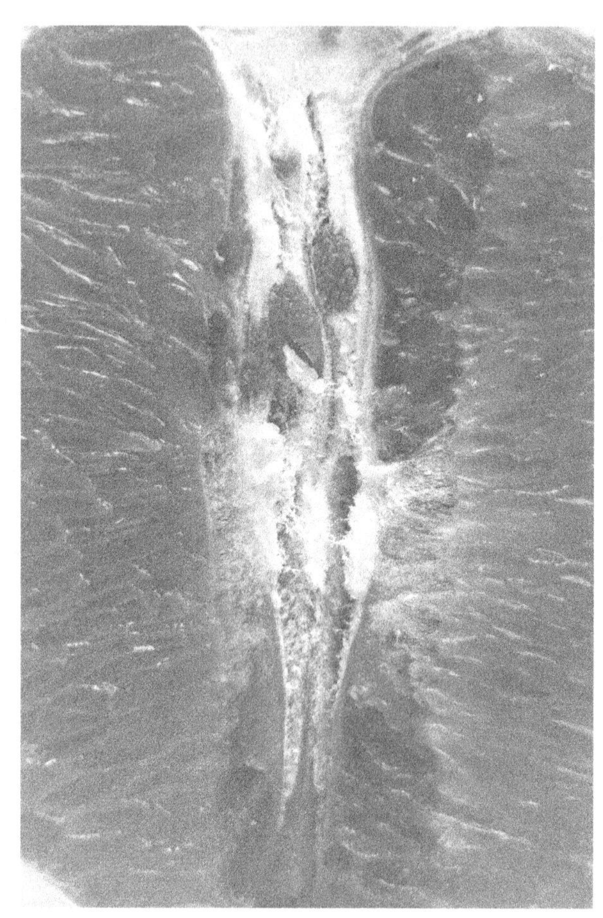

| GALVESTON COOKBOOK RECIPE

Introduction

Galveston Cuisine

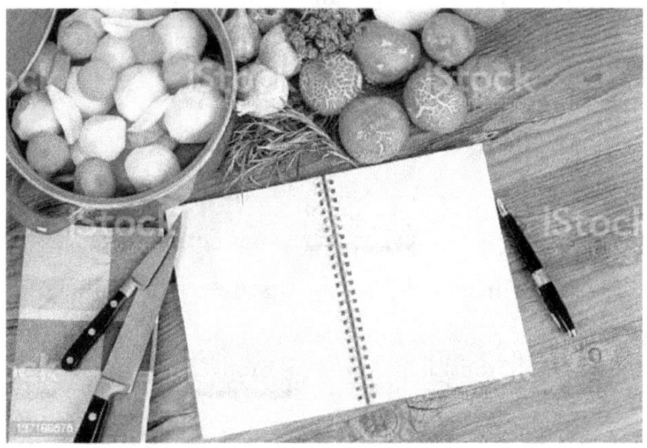

As you begin your culinary adventure through the "Galveston Cookbook," begin with "Introduction to Galveston Cuisine." Here, we immerse ourselves in the captivating realm of tastes that constitute Galveston's culinary culture.

Galveston's Flavors

Consider the salty air carrying whispers of the Gulf of Mexico, mixed with the earthy odors of fresh seafood and sun-ripened fruit. This section goes into the very core of Galveston's cuisine—a rare combination of sea and land.

These aromas are as varied as the island itself, ranging from the saline notes of Gulf shrimp to the strong spices of Tex-Mex.

Galveston Culinary History

Every dish includes a bit of Galveston's history. Discover the island's unique background as a thriving port city and how it inspired its culinary traditions. Discover how immigrant cultures, from Cajuns to Mexican migrants, have contributed to Galveston's unique culinary culture. You'll acquire a solid knowledge of the varied melting pot that is the food of this island.

Ingredients from the Region

This section looks into the riches of Galveston's land and waterways.

We identify the unique components that make Galveston cuisine genuinely one-of-a-kind, from Gulf Coast seafood like delicious shrimp and sweet crab to locally grown fruit like juicy Texas citrus and farm-fresh veggies.

You'll understand why Galveston's chefs employ the freshest, most genuine ingredients for their masterpieces.

 sets the scene for the gastronomic experience that awaits in the following chapters with each page turn.

 The Flavors of Galveston, its rich Culinary History, and the distinctive Ingredients will guide you as you discover the magnificent dishes and tales that make this excellent cookbook.

Prepare to be charmed by the spirit of Galveston's cuisine, which unites the sea, history, and tradition on your plate

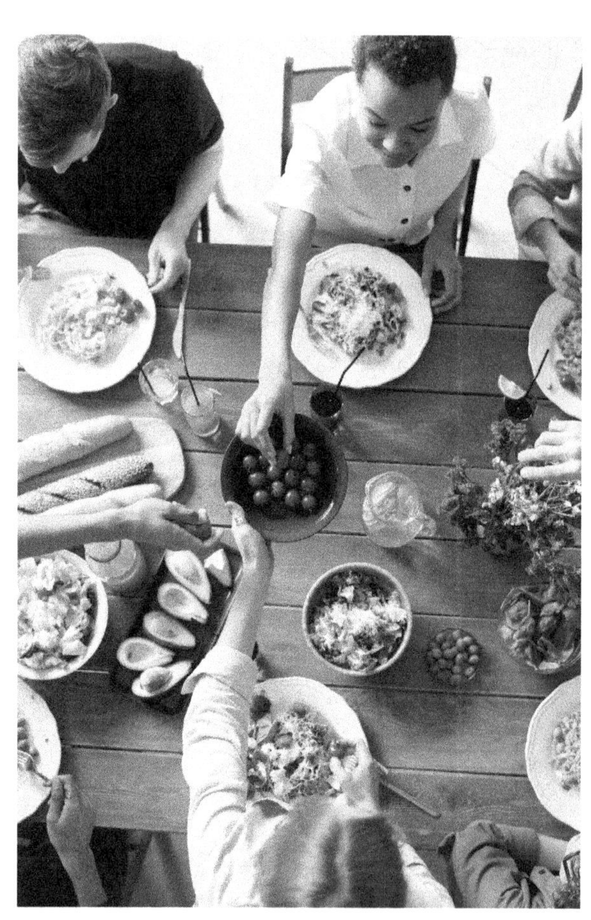

GALVESTON COOKBOOK RECIPE

The Flavors of Galveston

As you walk into the first subchapter, "The Flavors of Galveston," you'll find a sensory experience unlike any other in the "Galveston Cookbook." Here, we expose the essence of Galveston's culinary identity—a remarkable blend of sea and land, where vivid tastes mirror the island's dynamic spirit.

- ❖ **A Taste of the Gulf:** Salty Ocean Breezes

    Close your eyes and envision yourself standing on the beaches of Galveston Island, the salty Gulf of Mexico air caressing your face.

    Galveston's flavor starts here, with the best seafood available. The area is famed for its plump and delicious Gulf shrimp. Their saline flavor wonderfully reflects the character of the Gulf seas.

In this segment, you'll learn how to cook Gulf Shrimp Scampi, a meal where the natural tastes of the sea take center stage.

❖ **A Spice Symphony:** Tex-Mex and Southwestern Influences

Galveston's culinary landscape would be incomplete without a fiery embrace of Tex-Mex and Southwestern influences.

Spices that are bright, vivid, and fragrant add a unique flavor to dishes. Enchiladas Verdes with Roasted Salsa emphasizes the strength of chili peppers, the smokiness of cumin, and the diversity of tastes. Galveston's Tex-Mex past provides an interesting touch to the island's food, and you'll learn how to duplicate these distinct tastes in your own kitchen.

Land and Sea Bounty: Fusion at Its Finest

What actually differentiates Galveston is its culinary fusion expertise. Elements from the sea and the mainland mingle together to produce recipes that are both peaceful and interesting.

Imagine a meal that blends the freshness of Gulf redfish with the rich, powerful flavors of Creole cuisine: Blackened Redfish with Creole Sauce.

In Galveston, the tastes of land and sea mix to produce a gastronomic experience that is nothing short of amazing.

With each page in this area, you'll have a greater knowledge of the tastes that characterize Galveston cuisine.

Whether you're a seafood fanatic, a spice expert, or simply someone who appreciates the art of culinary fusion, "The Flavors of Galveston" will leave your taste buds tingling with excitement for the gourmet treats that await in the "Galveston Cookbook."

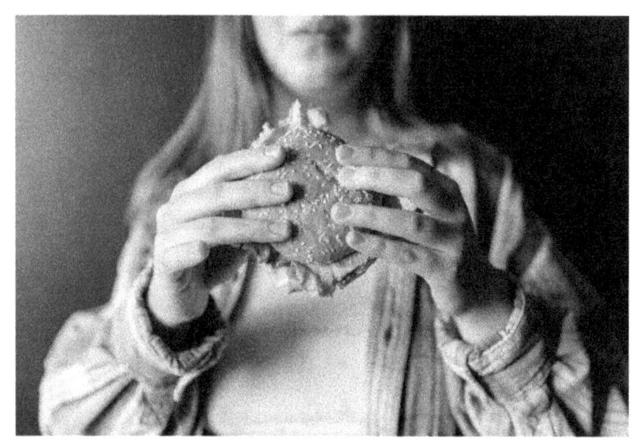

| GALVESTON COOKBOOK RECIPE

Culinary History of Galveston

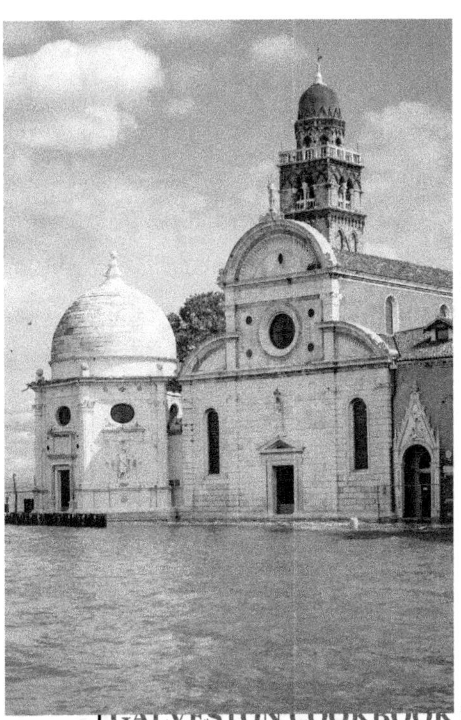

The second subchapter of "The Galveston Cookbook," "Culinary History of Galveston," provides a riveting description of how Galveston's culinary traditions have thrived, tied to the island's rich history, cultural influences, and culinary legacy.

- ❖ **Galveston's Maritime Influence:** Port City Origins Galveston called the "Wall Street of the South," was a bustling port city in the nineteenth century, playing a significant role in commerce, business, and immigration. This maritime background has a tremendous effect on its gastronomic heritage.

  Discover how many civilizations, seafarers, and merchants introduced a range of cuisines to the island. Galveston's early days laid the groundwork for a cuisine that would be indelibly defined by its naval background, from spices to exotic ingredients.

  A Taste of Louisiana with Cajun and Creole Influence Louisiana's culinary influence is abundantly visible in Galveston's cuisine. As you tour this area, you'll learn about the Cajun and Creole influences that have extended throughout the Gulf.

  Cajun Jambalaya with Andouille Sausage pays respect to these rich culinary traditions, showing the Creole cuisine's blend of French, African, and Spanish components. Galveston's Creole connection lends a spicy, savory aspect to the city's gastronomic culture.

❖ **Immigrant Communities:** A Multi-Flavor Tapestry Galveston's past is one of immigration and variety, which is reflected in its cuisine. Mexican settlers, Irish immigrants, and others brought their culinary traditions with them, producing a diverse tapestry of tastes.

Learn how these groups permeated the Galveston culinary tapestry with their diverse tastes, recipes, and habits. This chapter shows how immigrant groups have shaped Galveston's food, making it a location where every meal offers a tale of tradition and history. By the conclusion of "Culinary History of Galveston," you'll have a clear knowledge of how Galveston's history affects its contemporary culinary environment.

The tastes of the globe have blended and grown on this island, resulting in a diversified and delectable cuisine that pays tribute to the island's rich heritage.

This chapter sets the scene for the culinary experiences that await in the "Galveston Cookbook," where you'll

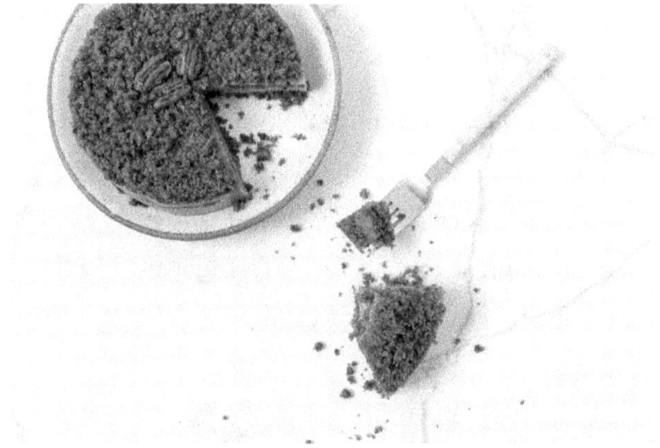

learn about this magnificent island's rich history.

Ingredients Unique to the Region

Prepare to embark on a gastronomic treasure hunt in the third subchapter of "The Galveston Cookbook," "Ingredients Unique to the Region." Here, we dig into the hidden jewels and tastes that distinguish Galveston's distinctive cuisine, exhibiting the island's vast variety.

- ❖ **Succulent Gulf Seafood:** Galveston's Heartbeat

  Close your eyes and envision the glittering waters of the Gulf of Mexico alive with life. Galveston's gastronomic character takes root here.

  From plump Gulf shrimp and Gulf Coast crab to flaky redfish and snapper, the Gulf has it all. These marine delicacies are the lifeblood of Galveston's cuisine, and you'll learn how to appreciate their natural tastes in dishes like Blackened Redfish with Creole Sauce and Galveston Bay Crab Cakes in this section.

❖ **Texas Citrus:** A Sunshine Burst

The climate in Galveston is great for producing citrus fruits that explode with taste and vitality. The spicy world of Texas citrus is explored in this part, from the acidic brightness of Ruby Red grapefruits to the delicate sweetness of Texas oranges.

These citrus beauties are typically used in pleasant drinks such as Tropical Fruit Smoothies, giving a bit of sunshine to your culinary creations.

❖ **Island Bounty:** Local Farm-Fresh Produce

The island's fertile soil and mild temperature also produce an abundance of fresh veggies and herbs. Galveston's chefs have long understood the significance of employing local, seasonal foods, and in this part, you'll learn how to cook meals that accentuate the island's agricultural background.

Taste the vibrant flavors of Galveston's soil by creating dishes like Farm-Fresh Vegetable Medley.

As you browse through the pages of this section, you'll develop a new admiration for the exquisite meals that grace Galveston's kitchens.

The Gulf seafood, Texas citrus, and local vegetables serve as the basis for the island's gourmet character. "Ingredients Unique to the Region" will encourage you to integrate these jewels into your own kitchen, enabling you to capture the essence of Galveston's cuisine in every meal.

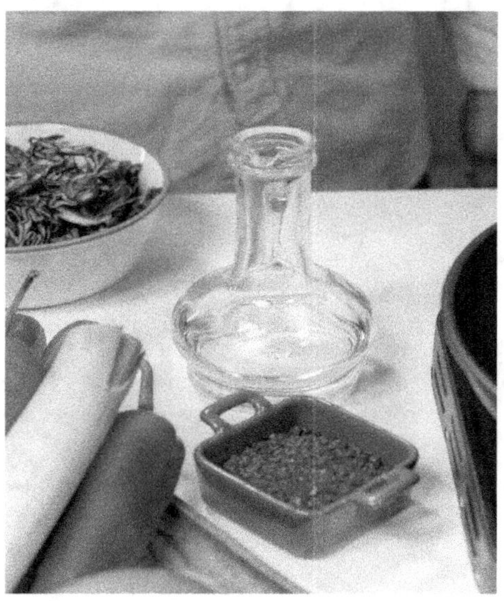

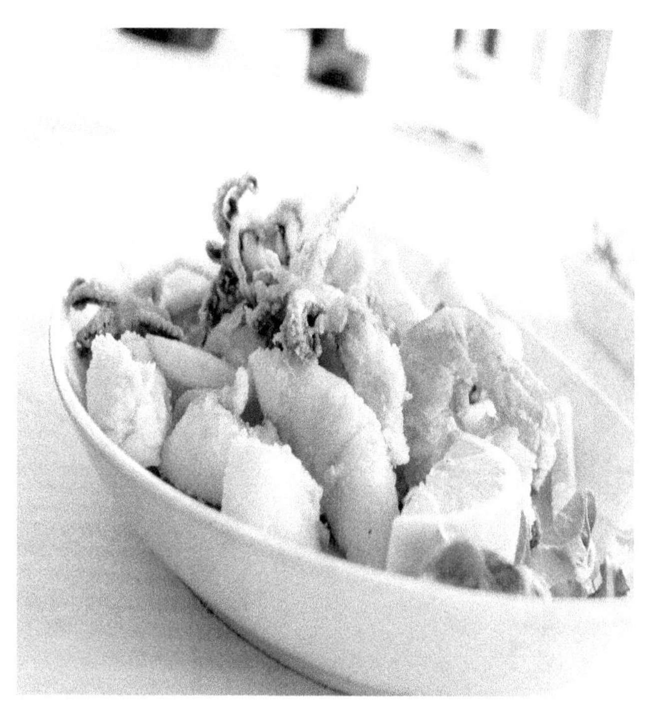

| GALVESTON COOKBOOK RECIPE

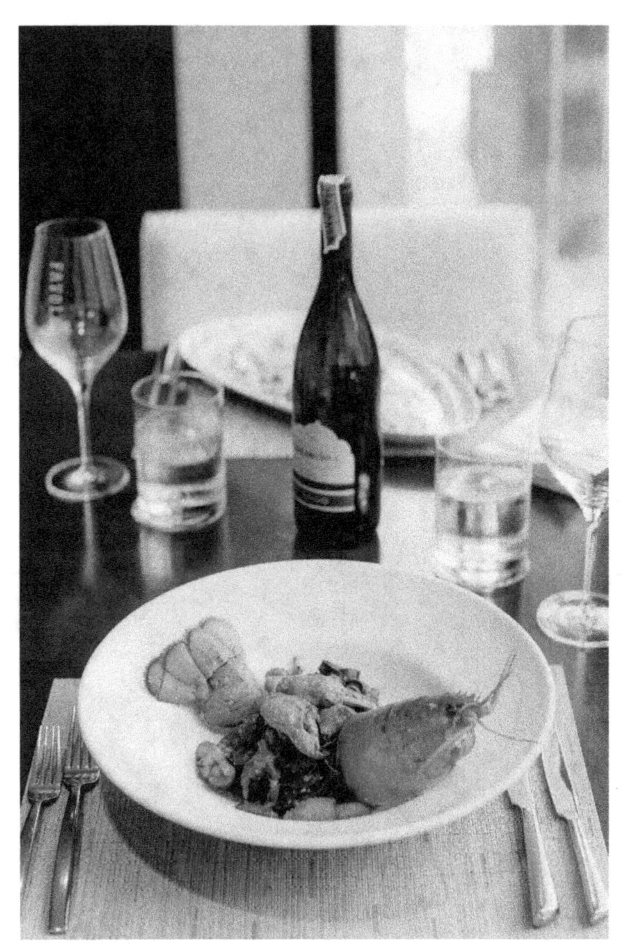

| GALVESTON COOKBOOK RECIPE

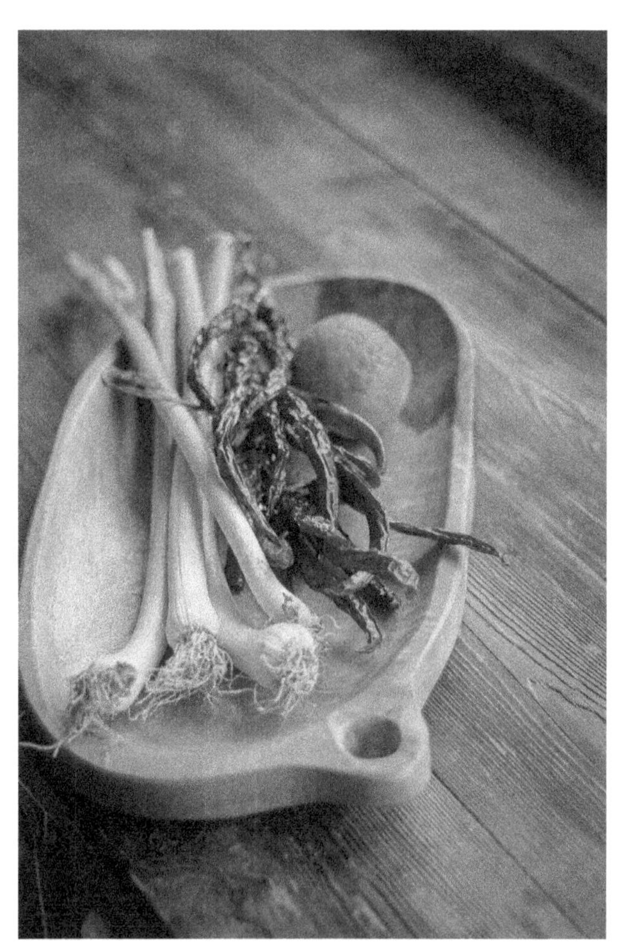

| GALVESTON COOKBOOK RECIPE

Chapter 1: Seafood Delights

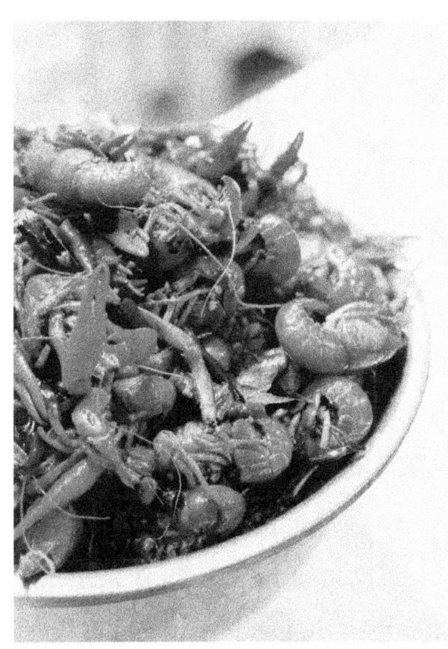

Prepare to embark on a culinary adventure as you dip into Chapter 2 of "The Galveston Cookbook" - "Seafood Delights." This chapter is a love letter to the Gulf of Mexico, where the finest seafood is converted into wonderful dinners that will drive your taste buds into a frenzy.

❖ **Fresh Gulf Shrimp Scampi:** A Flavor Symphony

Consider plump Gulf shrimp caressed by the sea wind and sautéed to perfection in a fragrant garlic and butter sauce. Each exquisite taste erupts with the flavor of Galveston's maritime charm.

 In this part, we explain the secrets to cooking Fresh Gulf Shrimp Scampi, a supper that epitomizes the essence of the Gulf seas. The shrimp take center stage in this symphony of flavors, with garlic, butter, and a hint of lemon providing the appropriate accompaniment.

A Crispy Tribute to the Gulf: Galveston Bay Crab Cakes

The Galveston Bay Crab Cakes exhibit Galveston's culinary abilities. Consider little bits of sweet crab flesh linked together with breadcrumbs and fragrant spices, then pan-fried to golden perfection.

These crab cakes pay respect to the island's seafaring past while highlighting the richness of the Gulf. You'll learn how to prepare these golden patties and how to infuse them with the particular tastes of Galveston.

❖ **A Spicy Gulf Adventure:** Blackened Redfish with Creole Sauce

Prepare to embark on a spicy adventure as you discover Blackened Redfish with Creole Sauce in this area. This meal is a Gulf cuisine masterpiece in which redfish is lavishly covered in a spicy blend of Cajun spices before being seared to develop a smokey covering.

It comes with a thick and tangy Creole sauce that provides a punch of flavor. Every taste tells a narrative about the Gulf's vibrant and varied culinary tradition.

The second chapter of "The Galveston Cookbook" is a sensory voyage over the Gulf's wonders.

You'll enjoy the flavor of Galveston's coastal cuisine, from the delicate delicacy of crab cakes to the fiery embrace of burned redfish.

Each dish evokes the essence of the sea and the island's profound connection to its nautical past. Prepare to be taken directly to the beaches of Galveston by seafood delicacies.

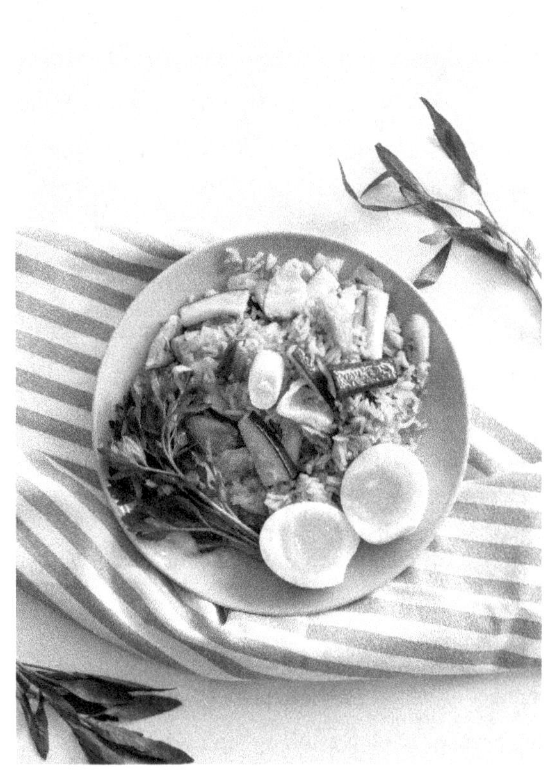

GALVESTON COOKBOOK RECIPE

Fresh Gulf Shrimp Scampi

In the heart of "Seafood Delights" inside "The Galveston Cookbook," there's an entire section devoted to the wonderful Fresh Gulf Shrimp Scampi—a culinary miracle that reflects the Gulf's marine bounty and Galveston's coastal charm.

- ❖ **The Gulf Shrimp Dance:** A Taste of the Sea

  Close your eyes and envision the magnificent, life-filled waters of the Gulf of Mexico. The centerpiece of this meal, the Gulf shrimp, rises from these blue depths. These plump, delectable shrimp, caressed by the sea wind, are at the core of Fresh Gulf Shrimp Scampi.

  Their sweet and briny tastes transport you to Galveston's sun-kissed beach.

- ❖ **Garlic and Butter's Fragrant Alchemy:** A Mediterranean Touch

  The natural sweetness of shrimp dances with the aromatic appeal of garlic and the creamy richness of butter in this delightful symphony of tastes. In this part, you'll discover how to infuse these components to produce a sauce that not only complements but lifts the shrimp to gourmet brilliance.

The perfumed garlic-butter bath meeting the sizzling shrimp is a gourmet treat unlike any other.

A Citrus Zest with a Lemon Hint

Fresh Gulf Shrimp Scampi embraces the fresh, citrusy scents of lemon to balance the richness of the butter and the savory garlic. This fruit's zest and juice give a refreshing and tart contrast, giving each mouthful a beautiful combination of tastes. The acidity of the lemon cuts through the richness of the meal, leaving a pleasant, long-lasting impact in your tongue.

Elegant Serving: Pairing and Presentation

In the culinary arts, presentation is essential, and this section will teach you how to plate Fresh Gulf Shrimp Scampi with elegance and flare.

You'll find the right way to serve this Gulf-inspired delicacy, whether it's over al dente pasta, a bed of fresh greens, or with crusty bread to soak up every drop of the rich sauce.

Fresh Gulf Shrimp Scampi is more than simply a supper; it's a salute to Galveston's seaside magnificence. It's a celebration of the Gulf's abundance and the island's lasting link to its marine past.

In this chapter, you'll discover how to produce a culinary masterpiece that represents the essence of Galveston's food, where the sea, garlic, butter, and lemon merge in a symphony of tastes that's nothing short of remarkable.

Galveston Bay Crab Cakes

In the heart of Galveston's coastal cuisine, buried between the pages of "The Galveston Cookbook," you'll discover a culinary masterpiece that, with every taste, recounts the story of Galveston's maritime heritage. Welcome to: "Galveston Bay Crab Cakes," where the riches of the Gulf are converted into golden, exquisite treats.

- ❖ **Golden Bounty of Galveston Bay:** Sweet Crab Meat Close your eyes and envision yourself on the sun-kissed beaches of Galveston Bay, where the peaceful lapping of the waves coincides with the harvest of sweet, exquisite crab flesh.

This dish pays tribute to the Gulf's golden bounty: gem-like morsels of crab flesh. Each taste reflects the spirit of Galveston's beachfront charm, a testimony to the island's longtime love affair with water.

❖ **A Symphony of Ingredients:** The Art of the Cake

Galveston Bay Crab Cakes are a superb culinary masterpiece. Consider a delicate combination of fresh crab flesh, breadcrumbs, mild spices, and a dollop of mayonnaise.

As a result, the mixture is delicately seasoned, correctly textured, and ready to be turned into golden patties. This course will teach you how to make magnificent cakes with the precision and artistry they deserve.

Golden Brown and Crispy Pan-Fried Perfection

As you begin on your culinary journey, you'll learn the key to attaining the ideal texture: pan-frying. Watch as the crab cakes sizzle in a hot skillet, their exteriors turning golden brown and wonderfully crispy while the insides stay supple and savory. The symphony of sizzling, the perfume of toasted breadcrumbs, and the anticipation of the first taste combine to offer an experience that is beyond ordinary cooking.

❖ **A Burst of Gulf Flavor:** Galveston's Essence

Each mouthful of a Galveston Bay Crab Cake tells a narrative—a tale of the Gulf's bounty, the island's respect for its nautical heritage, and the culinary expertise that elevates basic ingredients into a gourmet masterpiece. These crab cakes, whether served as an appetizer, a main entrée, or a side dish, are a tribute to Galveston's devotion to honoring its maritime past.

Galveston Bay Crab Cakes are more than just a meal; they're a love letter to Galveston, a testament to the city's everlasting love affair with the sea, and an invitation to wallow in the Gulf's treasures in all their golden magnificence.

This chapter encourages you to learn how to produce these wonderful dishes so that your dining experience reflects the real taste of Galveston's beach cuisine.

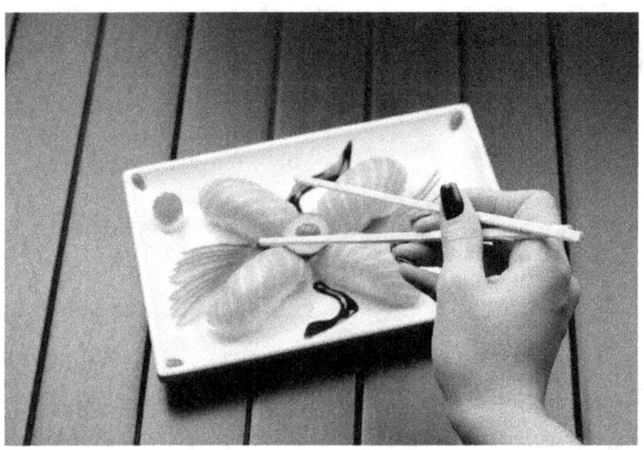

Blackened Redfish with Creole Sauce

Prepare to travel on a fiery, flavor-filled voyage into the

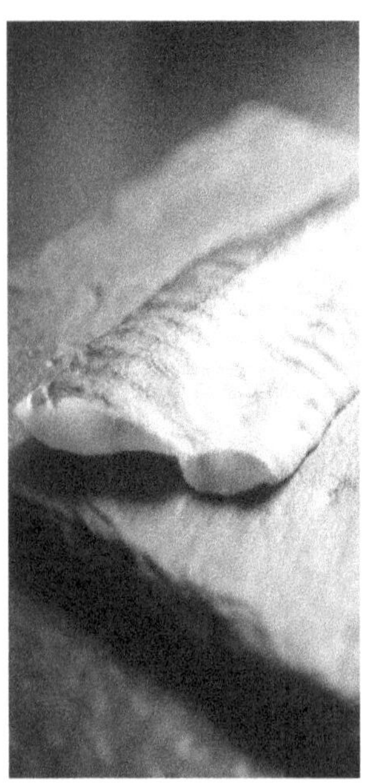

heart of Galveston's culinary tradition as you plunge into "The Galveston Cookbook"—"Blackened Redfish with Creole Sauce." This recipe reflects the essence of Gulf cuisine, mixing the robust, spicy tastes of the Gulf with a hint of Creole refinement.

❖ **Redfish:** A Gulf Specialty

Consider the calm Gulf waters, where redfish flourish in the sun-dappled waves. The stars of our meal are these crimson-hued beauties, noted for their crisp, flaky texture and rich, intense taste.

The usage of redfish is no accident; it is a monument to Galveston's devotion to presenting the Gulf's greatest resources in its culinary creations.

A Fiery Cajun Blend of Blackened Magic

The alchemy of spice is embraced in this culinary masterpiece of charred redfish. Cajun-inspired seasoning, a combination of spicy paprika, cayenne pepper, thyme, and other fragrant spices, turns this meal into a flavor symphony.

As you move through this phase, you'll learn how to apply the blackening spices to the redfish, resulting in a smoky crust that tantalizes the fish's intrinsic richness.

Zesty and Flavorful Creole Sauce

The centerpiece of this meal is the Creole sauce. Consider a rich, tangy tomato-based sauce combined with the vibrant taste of Creole cuisine. It's a rich and colorful sauce created from sour tomatoes, fragrant herbs, and a variety of spices.

As you go through the recipe, you'll find the elements to preparing a Creole sauce that compliments the blackened redfish.

❖ **A Culinary Symphony:** The Marriage of Flavors

The mix of tastes is what makes Blackened Redfish with Creole Sauce so wonderful. The blackened redfish's smokey, peppery crust meets the creamy, zesty embrace of the Creole sauce.

It's a gourmet ballet in which each swallow is a burst of adrenaline, a crescendo of sensations that tingle your taste receptors. It's a meal that epitomizes the vibrant, variegated character of Gulf cuisine.

"The Galveston Cookbook" Chapter 1 encourages you to experience the miracle of Blackened Redfish with Creole Sauce, where the richness of the Gulf meets the dramatic history of Creole cuisine.

As you begin on this adventure, you will not only learn how to cook this renowned meal, but you will also receive a deep understanding of Galveston's particular culinary culture—a culture that feeds on the marriage of tastes, the essence of the Gulf, and the zest of Creole lineage.

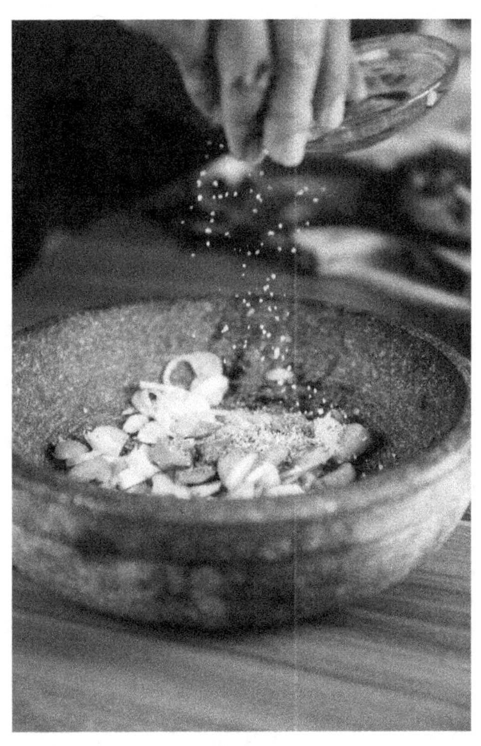

GALVESTON COOKBOOK RECIPE

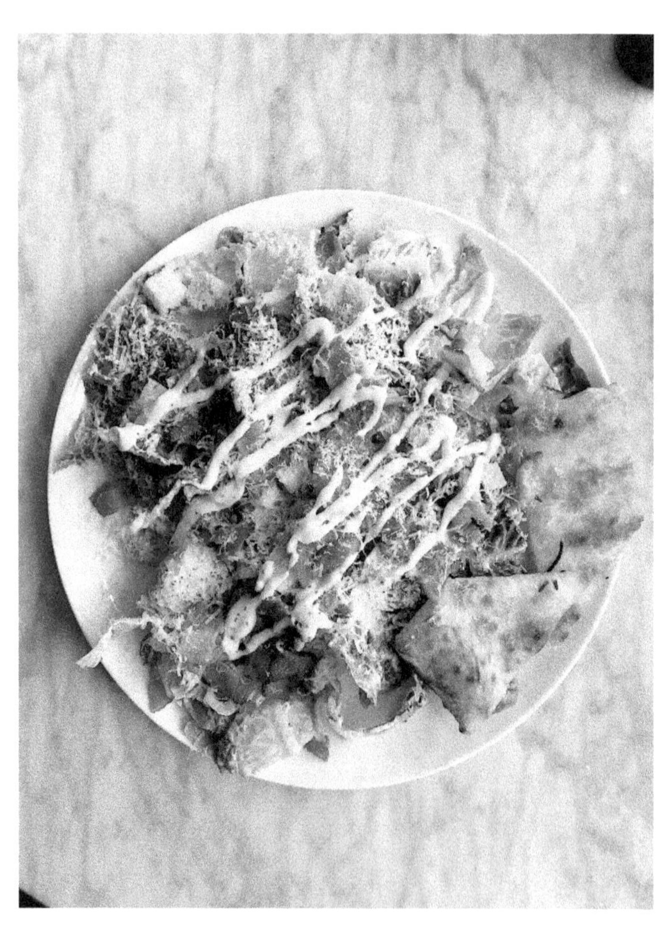

| GALVESTON COOKBOOK RECIPE

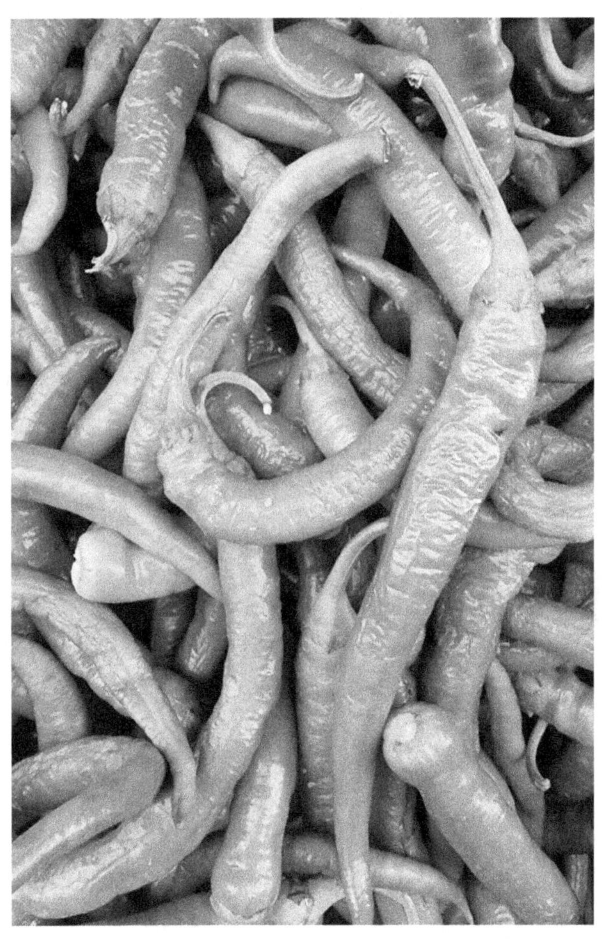

| GALVESTON COOKBOOK RECIPE

Chapter 2: Tex-Mex and Southwestern Influences

Welcome to a chapter bursting to the seams with brilliant colors, robust tastes, and a blazing passion for Tex-Mex and Southwestern cuisine. In Chapter 2 of "The Galveston Cookbook," we travel on an exciting culinary excursion into the heart of Galveston, where the confluence of Tex-Mex and Southwestern influences results in tantalizing meals.

- ❖ **Spicy Galveston Chili:** A Comforting Tex-Mex Classic

  Expect to be surrounded by the fragrance of boiling chili—a Tex-Mex classic—in this region. This traditional meal is given a marine touch in Galveston by combining Gulf seafood and a combination of spices that stimulate the tongue.

  Each mouthful is a flavor explosion, with earthy beans, scorching chiles, and exquisite fish. You'll learn how to cook Spicy Galveston Chili, a supper that warms the spirit while paying respect to the aggression of Tex-Mex cuisine.

Southwestern Enchiladas Verdes with Roasted Salsa

As we continue through this chapter, we come across the fascinating world of Enchiladas Verdes—a Southwestern masterpiece. Consider soft tortillas wrapped around a delectable filling and bathed in a brilliant green salsa prepared from roasted tomatillos and chiles. The outcome is a meal that is both beautiful and tasty. This

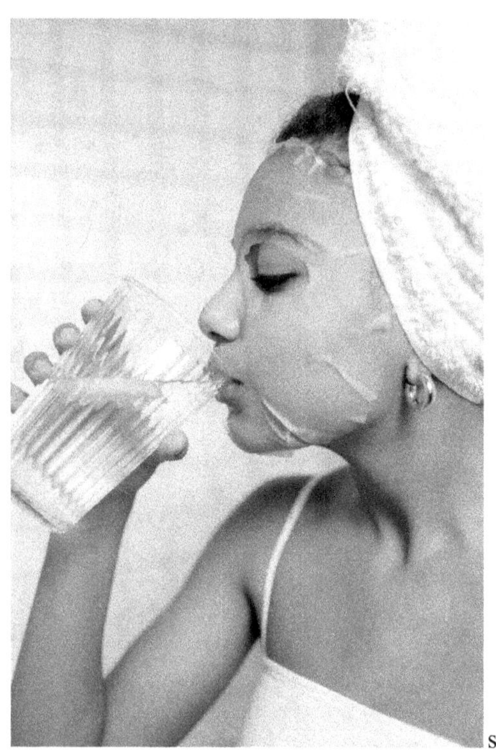

section leads you through the specific stages of cooking Enchiladas Verdes with Roasted Salsa, a Southwestern-inspired cuisine.

Flavor Fiesta Tex-Mex Tacos with Homemade Tortillas

Our journey would not be complete without a visit to the Tex-Mex taco seller.

You'll learn how to prepare Tex-Mex Tacos with Homemade Tortillas right here. Consider soft, pillowy tortillas encasing your favorite filling, such as luscious grilled prawns or smokey pork. Add a colorful variety of toppings, such as fresh salsa and creamy guacamole, and you've got a Tex-Mex feast that's a gourmet carnival for the senses.

This section leads you through the complete process, from preparing your own tortillas to creating your own taco.

"The Galveston Cookbook" Chapter 2 allows you to savor the rich and dynamic flavors of Tex-Mex and Southwestern cuisine, a reflection of the blazing passion that distinguishes Galveston's culinary environment. Each meal is a celebration of the combination of spices, the art of presentation, and the region's rich cultural tapestry.

 By the conclusion of this chapter, you'll be able to make these

Tex-Mex and Southwestern favorites in your own

kitchen, enabling you to taste the lively flavor of Galveston's

food wherever you are.

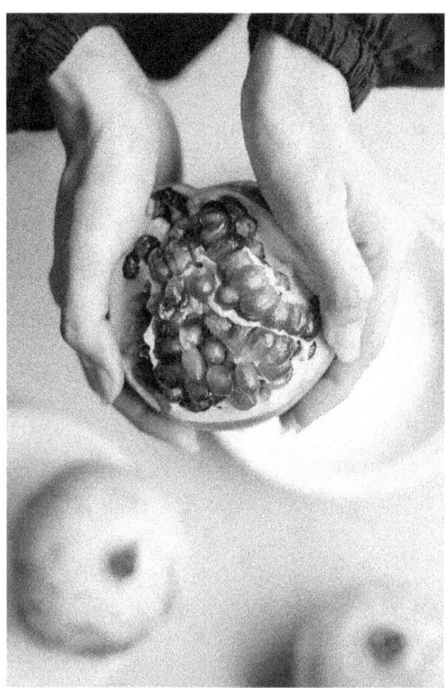

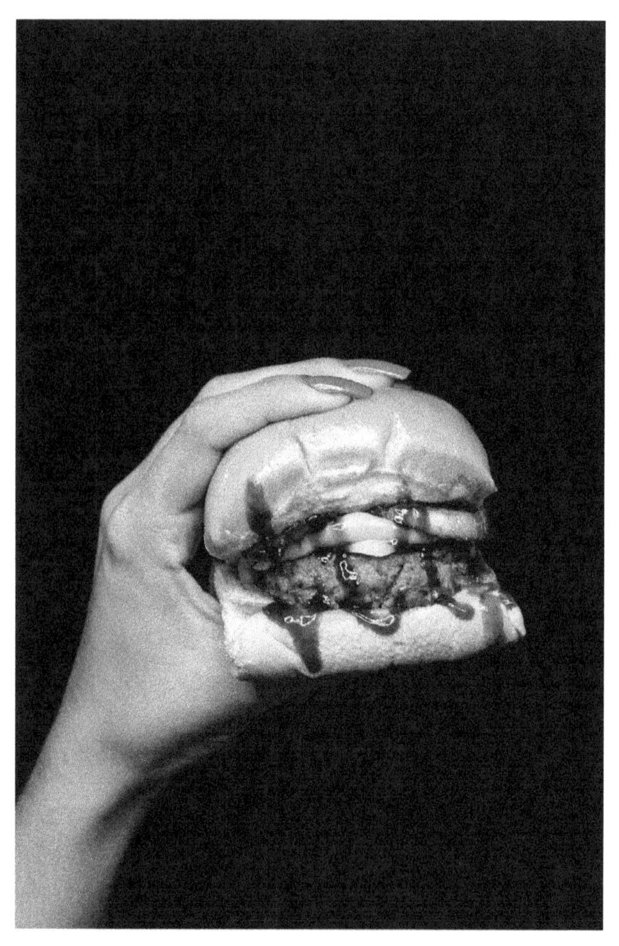

| GALVESTON COOKBOOK RECIPE

Spicy Galveston Chili

Prepare your taste buds for a terrific Tex-Mex trip as we dig into Chapter 2 of "The Galveston Cookbook" - "Spicy Galveston Chili." This recipe is a robust celebration of tastes, blending the warmth of chili with the nautical flare of Galveston's Gulf seafood.

A Traditional Tex-Mex Dish with a Gulf Twist

Consider a warm pot of chili simmering on the stove, loaded with a wonderful assortment of ingredients. Spicy Galveston Chili takes the Tex-Mex staple to a whole new level by integrating the richness of the Gulf.

Plump shrimp, juicy crab flesh, and soft fish blend with classic chili components such as beans and fragrant spices. As a result, the meal is as substantial as it is vibrant—a perfect expression of Galveston's culinary flair.

❖ **The Art of Spices:** A Flavor Symphony

In this class, you'll learn about the method of spices, which is crucial in Tex-Mex cuisine. Chili powder, cumin, paprika, and cayenne pepper infuse the chili with rich, smokey flavors.

Each spice adds depth and complexity to the meal, producing a symphony of tastes that dance on your tongue. You'll learn how to blend these spices to create the right degree of heat and warmth in your Spicy Galveston Chili.

The Gulf Ingredients Shine in The Seafood Bounty

Spicy Galveston Chili is known for its all-star seafood cuisine. The delicious sweetness of Gulf shrimp balances the savory overtones of crab meat and the flaky texture of fish.

These spices offer a distinct coastal fragrance to the chili, bringing you to the beaches of Galveston with each taste.

Tex-Mex Feast with Garnishes and Sides

No Tex-Mex chili is complete without a range of exquisite garnishes and side dishes. In this segment, you'll learn how to cook a Tex-Mex feast using items like grated cheese, sour cream, and fresh cilantro.

Combine your chili with homemade cornbread or tortilla chips for a full meal that truly embraces Tex-Mex culinary tradition. Galveston is fiery. Chili is more than simply a meal; it shows Galveston's strong personality and love of the sea.

By the conclusion of this segment, you'll have the skills to produce this scrumptious masterpiece in your own house, enabling you to savor the Tex-Mex and Gulf Coast flavors that make Galveston's food so distinctive.

Enchiladas Verdes with Roasted Salsa

Prepare to be taken to the amazing world of Southwestern cuisine as we explore Chapter 2 of "The Galveston Cookbook" - "Enchiladas Verdes with Roasted Salsa. " This meal is a culinary marvel, blending the robust tastes of the Southwest with the charm of Galveston's seaside appeal.

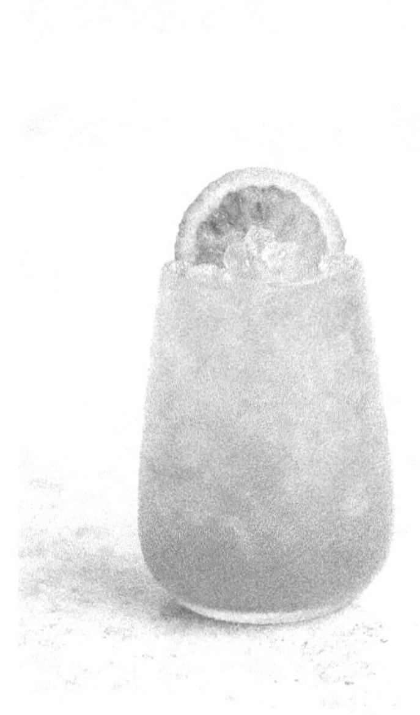

❖ **Enchiladas Verdes:** A Mexican Classic

Consider delicate tortillas that have been carefully packed with a delightful combination and then soaked in brilliant green salsa.

These are Enchiladas Verdes, a Southwestern staple that is as good as it is historical. This section will take you on a culinary trip through the process of producing Enchiladas Verdes, converting basic elements into a delicious symphony.

❖ **The Roasted Salsa:** The Dish's Heart

The Roasted Salsa serves as the meal's basis, a green elixir overflowing with the smokey smells of roasted tomatillos, the fire of green chilies, and the freshness of cilantro.

The salsa provides a fiery, acidic depth to the enchiladas, taking them to a gourmet level of complexity. You'll learn how to roast and blend the ingredients to produce a colorful and nuanced salsa that will make each taste an amazing experience.

Enchiladas Verdes are a blank canvas for your ideas. Fillings may range from soft shredded chicken to scrumptious grilled shrimp, and in this part, you'll learn how to produce the right filling.

Whether you choose to employ classic components or attempt something new, you'll learn how to infuse your enchiladas with tastes that match your culinary flair.

Showcase: Elegance Meets Flavor

Enchiladas Verde's presentation is an art form. You'll play with the presentation by garnishing with fresh cilantro, crumbled queso fresco, and a dollop of Mexican crema.

As a result, the supper is as aesthetically gorgeous as it is delicious—a feast for both the eyes and the mouth.

Enchiladas Verdes with Roasted Salsa is more than simply a supper; it's a study of Southwestern elegance and Galveston's passion for robust tastes.

By the conclusion of this segment, you'll be able to make a culinary masterpiece that symbolizes the essence of both worlds—a dinner that's both informal and exquisite, allowing you to appreciate the combination of Southwestern and coastal flavors that characterize Galveston's gastronomy.

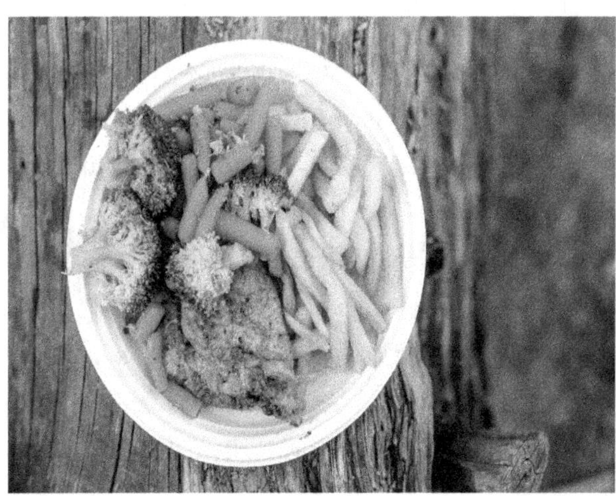

Tex-Mex Tacos with Homemade Tortillas

Welcome to a Tex-Mex feast inside "The Galveston Cookbook." In Chapter 2 we enter into the wonderful world of "Tex-Mex Tacos with Homemade Tortillas." This is where the passion of Tex-Mex meets the innovation of creating your own tortillas from scratch.

❖ **Tex-Mex Tacos:** An Explosion of Flavor

Consider a bright tray full of tacos, each a bite-sized explosion of taste. Tex-Mex Tacos are a prized culinary legacy, and in this part, you'll learn how to cook these gorgeous treats.

The filling possibilities are as diverse as your taste buds, ranging from exquisite grilled prawns to smokey beef. The homemade tortilla, on the other hand, is the star of the show—a canvas for taste, texture, and authenticity.

❖ **From Dough to Delight:** The Art of Tortilla Making Homemade tortillas are the heart and soul of Tex-Mex tacos, and this section leads you through the process of creating them.

   You'll learn how to create a basic but magical dough out of flour, water, and a touch of salt. As you spread out the dough and fry it on a hot griddle, you'll watch how these simple components change into soft, pillowy tortillas—the ideal carrier for your Tex-Mex meals.

❖ **Tex-Mex Toppings:** A Flavorful Feast
The charm of Tex-Mex Tacos is found not only in the tortillas but also in the vibrant assortment of toppings and decorations. Each topping, from fresh salsa to creamy guacamole, adds layers of taste and texture.
The dish is concluded with crumbled queso fresco, shredded lettuce, and a squeeze of lime. This section will help you build the ultimate Tex-Mex taco, with

each mouthful a harmonic combination of tastes and textures.

❖ **Crafted with Love:** The Perfect Taco

Making Tex-Mex Tacos from scratch is a labor of love. It's about taking the time to produce something extraordinary, from the dough that transforms into tortillas to the precise assembling of each taco.

As a result, the taco becomes a gourmet experience, a celebration of the talent and passion that distinguish Tex-Mex cooking.

urges you to immerse yourself in the Tex-Mex culture, which mixes taste, heritage, and workmanship. By the conclusion of this session, you'll be able to produce Tex-Mex Tacos that show your love of robust tastes, respect for authenticity, and desire to savor the fusion of Tex-Mex traditions and

Galveston's culinary flare.

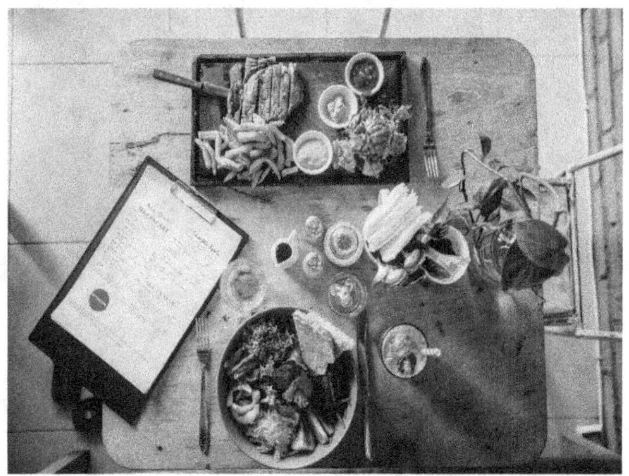

| GALVESTON COOKBOOK RECIPE

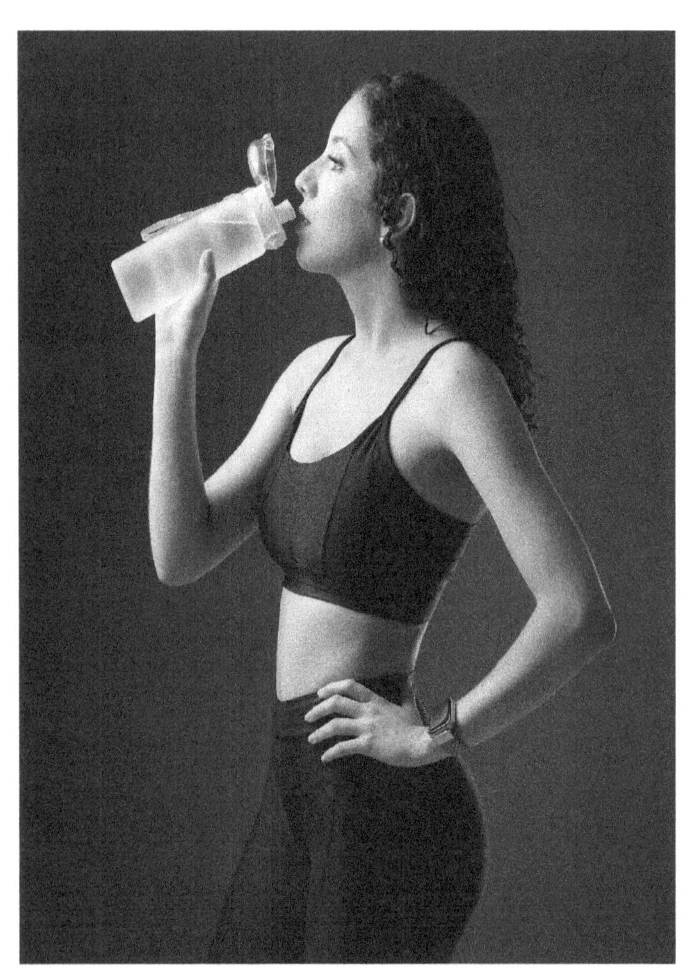

GALVESTON COOKBOOK RECIPE

Chapter 3: Southern Comfort Food

We immerse ourselves in the warm embrace of Southern Comfort Food in Chapter 3 of "The Galveston Cookbook," a gourmet voyage through meals that heal the soul.

This chapter is an homage to the rich legacy of comfort food, with each dish presenting a narrative of tradition, family, and good nights.

- ❖ **A Southern Classic:** Chicken and Waffles

   In this segment, we pay homage to a cherished Southern classic: Chicken and Waffles. Consider delicate, crispy fried chicken placed with fluffy, golden waffles topped with sweet maple syrup.

   It's a rich and comforting mixture, and you'll learn how to create it with a touch of Galveston's culinary flair.

- ❖ **A Coastal Delight:** Shrimp and Grits

   Our culinary trip continues with a seaside treat: Shrimp and Grits. Consider plump Gulf shrimp nestled above a bed of creamy, buttery grits and drizzled in a rich, delicious sauce.

This meal recalls Galveston's seafood history, where the richness of the Gulf meets the heartiness of Southern comfort.

❖ **Texas BBQ Brisket:** A Tasty Tradition

A taste of Texas BBQ Brisket would cap out any tour of comfort food. This section will introduce you to the world of slow-cooked, smokey brisket, which is tender, tasty, and a real Texas staple.

Discover the secrets to preparing luscious BBQ brisket that melts in your mouth by studying the art of smoking and seasoning.

❖ **Pecan Pie:** Sweet Southern Reminiscence

This chapter finishes with a taste of Sweet Southern Nostalgia—Pecan Pie. Consider a buttery, flaky crust filled with a delightful, gooey blend of nuts, brown sugar, and rich molasses.

It's a dinner as snug as a warm embrace and as sweet as treasured memories. This section will help you bake the ideal pecan pie, a piece of Southern bliss.

takes you deep into the heart of Southern Comfort Food, where each meal pays respect to the power of food to offer comfort, pleasure, and a feeling of belonging.

By the conclusion of this chapter, you'll not only know how to create these legendary dishes, but you'll also have a strong appreciation for the nostalgia, history, and warmth that Southern comfort food represents—a cuisine that greets you with open arms and a full meal.

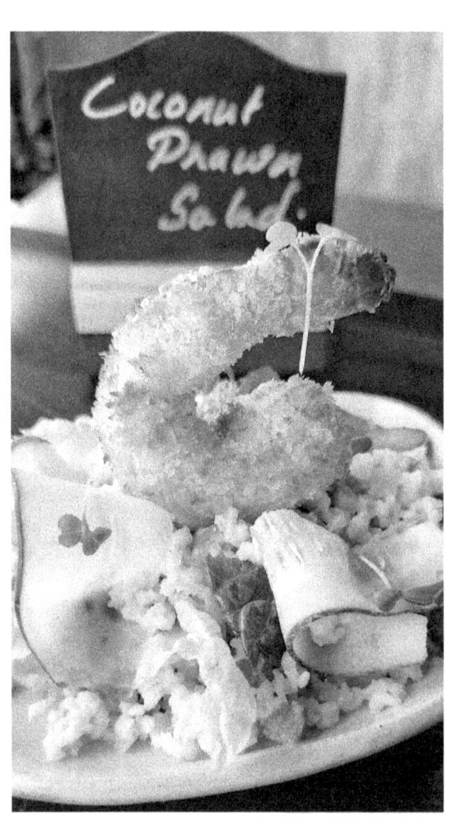
Coconut
Prawn
Salad

Chicken Fried Steak with Cream Gravy

As we explore Chapter 3 of "The Galveston Cookbook," "Chicken Fried Steak with Cream Gravy," we will reach the essence of comfort food nirvana.

This delectable and soul-satisfying traditional Southern meal epitomizes the spirit of comfort.

Chicken Fried Steak, a Hearty Southern Classic

Consider a plate heaped high with a golden, crispy steak that has been expertly seasoned and cooked to stunning perfection. This is the major component of Chicken Fried Steak.

In this part, we'll guide you through the process of cooking this favorite Southern cuisine. You'll learn how to prepare a wonderful coating that transforms an average steak into a crispy, savory masterpiece.

- ❖ **The Silky Elixir:** Cream Gravy

    But what is Chicken Fried Steak without the creamy accompaniment? The cream gravy is the recipe's crowning beauty, a silky elixir that envelops the steak in a rich, savory taste.

This part will show you how to prepare smooth, silky, and seductive cream gravy. Each pour over your sizzling steak is like a warm embrace for your taste receptors.

The Presentation and Sides of Southern Comfort

Comfort food is about more than simply the flavor; it's also about the experience. You'll learn about the art of presenting and delivering in this chapter.

You'll learn how to offer Chicken Fried Steak with Cream Gravy in an aesthetically attractive and welcoming approach. Don't forget the sides, such as mashed potatoes, collard greens, or buttered biscuits, which are designed to complement and improve the traditional experience.

❖ **Southern Hospitality on a Plate:** A Taste of Home Chicken Fried Steak with Cream Gravy is more than just a meal; it's a taste of home, a bit of Southern hospitality on a platter.

By the conclusion of this part, you'll not only have the skills to cook this traditional supper, but also a profound appreciation for the tradition, warmth, and emotional comfort that each mouthful provides—a dish that speaks to the soul and produces the impression of being enveloped in a warm, delicious embrace.

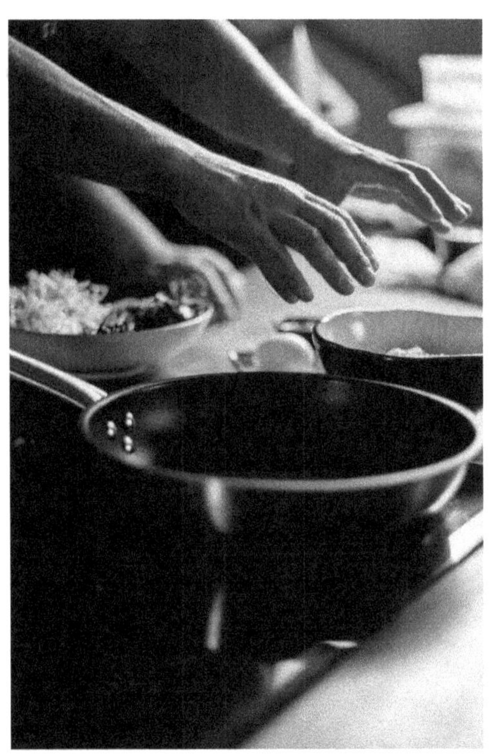

| GALVESTON COOKBOOK RECIPE

Buttermilk Biscuits and Sausage Gravy

In Chapter 3 of "The Galveston Cookbook," we get to the heart of Southern comfort cuisine with the timeless and delightful duet of "Buttermilk Biscuits and Sausage Gravy." This recipe is a symphony of flavors, a celebration of simplicity, and a soul-satisfying comfort food staple.

❖ **Pillowy Clouds of Comfort:** Buttermilk Biscuits Consider fresh-baked soft, flaky biscuits with a golden-brown top and a melt-in-your-mouth center. Buttermilk Biscuits are a Southern classic noted for their relaxing, buttery sweetness.

This chapter will show you how to create these pillowy clouds of happiness from scratch. From the preparation of the dough to the right baking procedure, you'll discover the secrets of producing smooth and tasty biscuits.

Rich and Satisfying Sausage Gravy

But what are Buttermilk Biscuits if not smothered in Sausage Gravy? This creamy, flavorful gravy is the ideal complement, a rich and delicious feature that elevates this meal to the next level. You'll learn how to prepare sausage gravy from scratch, with tastes like perfectly browned sausage, fragrant herbs, and creamy richness. Each mouthful is a flavor of Southern comfort.

❖ **The Art of Assembly:** Putting Everything Together
Southern comfort cuisine is about more than merely the individual components; it's about the satisfaction of combining them. In this part, you'll learn about the skill of assembly.

Consider a warm biscuit split in half and topped with a scoop of boiling hot sausage gravy. The biscuits soak up the creamy richness, providing a beautiful combination of textures and tastes.

❖ **A Southern Tradition:** Comfort on a Plate
Buttermilk Biscuits & Sausage Gravy is more than merely a meal; it's a taste of Southern history, a warm

embrace on a plate that invokes nostalgic sentiments, family reunions, and treasured memories.

By the conclusion of this segment, you'll not only have mastered the procedure for creating this traditional cuisine, but you'll also have a profound appreciation for the warmth, simplicity, and soul-satisfying delight it provides—food that warms the heart and fills the belly with Southern hospitality.

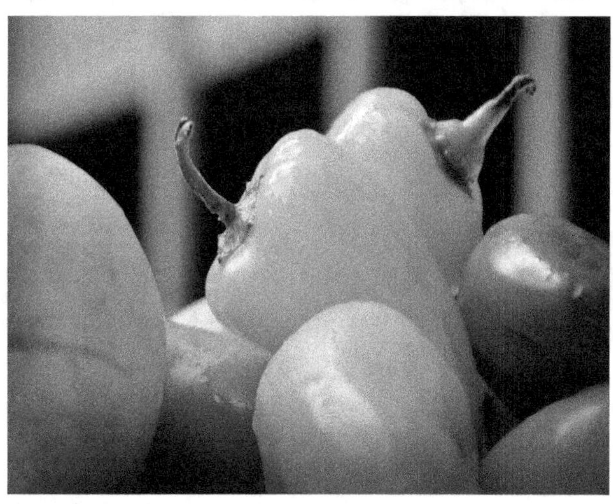

Cajun Jambalaya with Andouille Sausage

In Chapter 3 of "The Galveston Cookbook," we'll take a delectable vacation to the heart of Louisiana's culinary culture with "Cajun Jambalaya with Andouille Sausage." This recipe is a vivid and fragrant celebration of Cajun cuisine that will take your taste senses to the bayous of Louisiana.

- ❖ **Jambalaya:** A Culinary Fusion

    Jambalaya is a culinary melting pot of French, Spanish, African, and Caribbean components that highlights Louisiana's diverse cultural heritage. Consider a cast-iron pot simmering with a fragrant blend of rice, spicy Andouille sausage, succulent chicken, and aromatic veggies and spices.

    In this course, you'll dig into the art of cooking Jambalaya, exploring how to fill each grain of rice with a symphony of flavors.

    The Spicy and Smoky Essence of Andouille Sausage

Andouille sausage, a mainstay of Cajun cuisine, lies at the center of Jambalaya. This spicy and smoky sausage provides a robust and zesty flavor to the meal.

Learn how to pick, prepare, and cook Andouille sausage to perfection, ensuring that every mouthful is a flavor explosion.

❖ **Aromatic Harmony:** The Cajun Cooking Trinity

Cajun cuisine is recognized for its use of aromatic ingredients, and this part comprises the Trinity of Cajun cooking—a blend of onions, bell peppers, and celery.

This aromatic trio serves as the flavor basis for Jambalaya, resulting in a fragrant and savory base. The procedure of flawlessly sautéing these veggies is vital to attaining the dish's depth of flavor.

Presentation and Tradition in Serving a Taste of Louisiana

Jambalaya is more than simply a meal; it's anemblem of Louisiana's rich culture. You'll also learn about the art of presentation and tradition in this chapter.

Learn how to add color and freshness to your Jambalaya by garnishing it with fresh herbs such as chopped green onions and parsley.

Recognize the cultural importance of Jambalaya as a community food, commonly consumed during gatherings and holidays in Louisiana.

Cajun Jambalaya with Andouille Sausage is a culinary experience that immerses you in the tastes and traditions of Cajun cuisine. By the conclusion of this segment, you'll have mastered the process of cooking.

Jambalaya which captures the essence of Louisiana's bayous and embraces the dynamic spirit of this distinctive and memorable cuisine—a feast that's more than just food but a cultural experience.

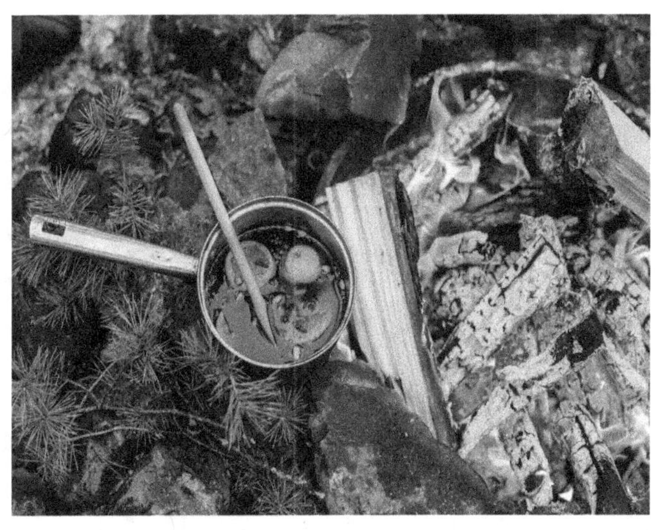

| GALVESTON COOKBOOK RECIPE

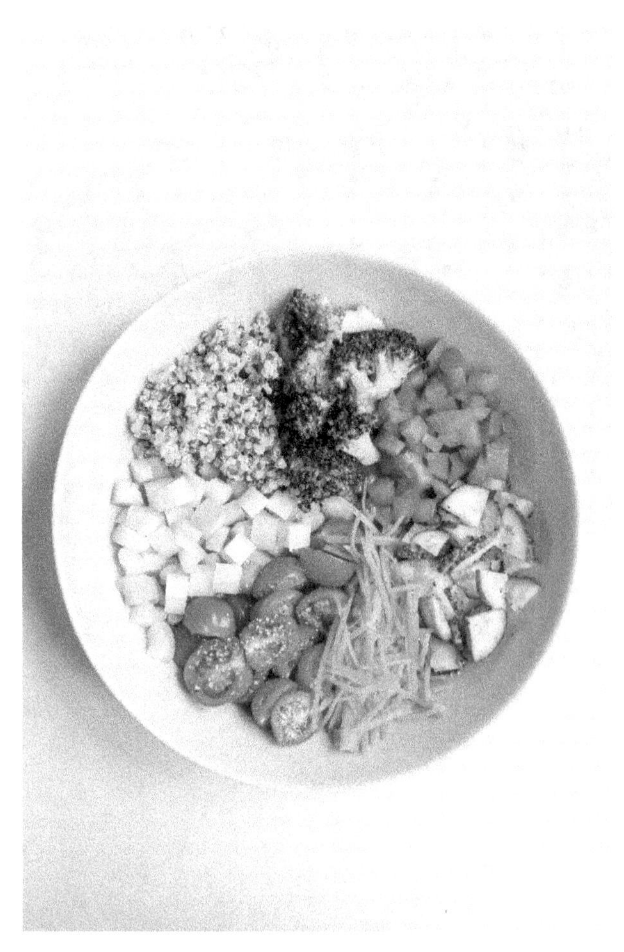

GALVESTON COOKBOOK RECIPE

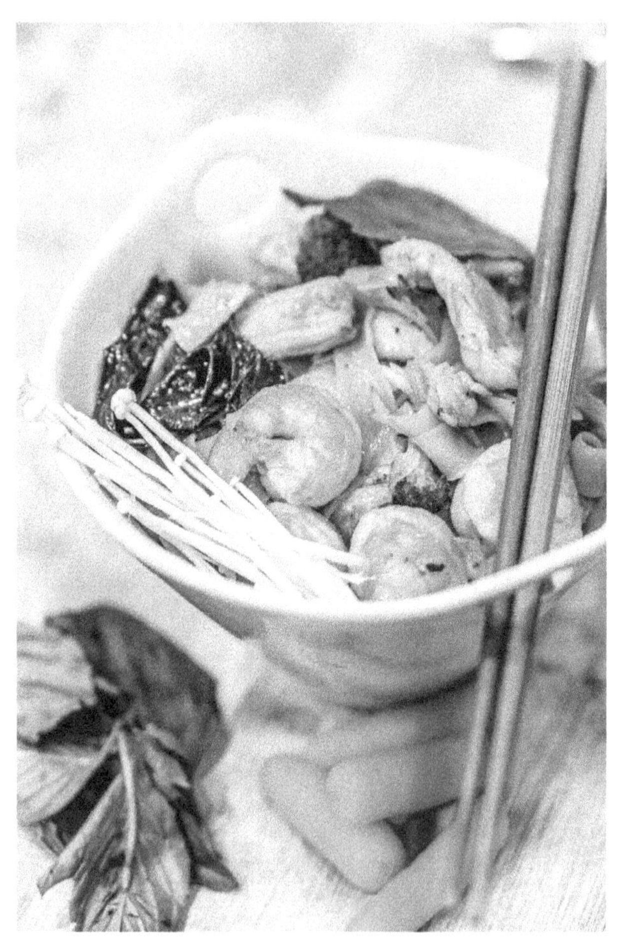

GALVESTON COOKBOOK RECIPE

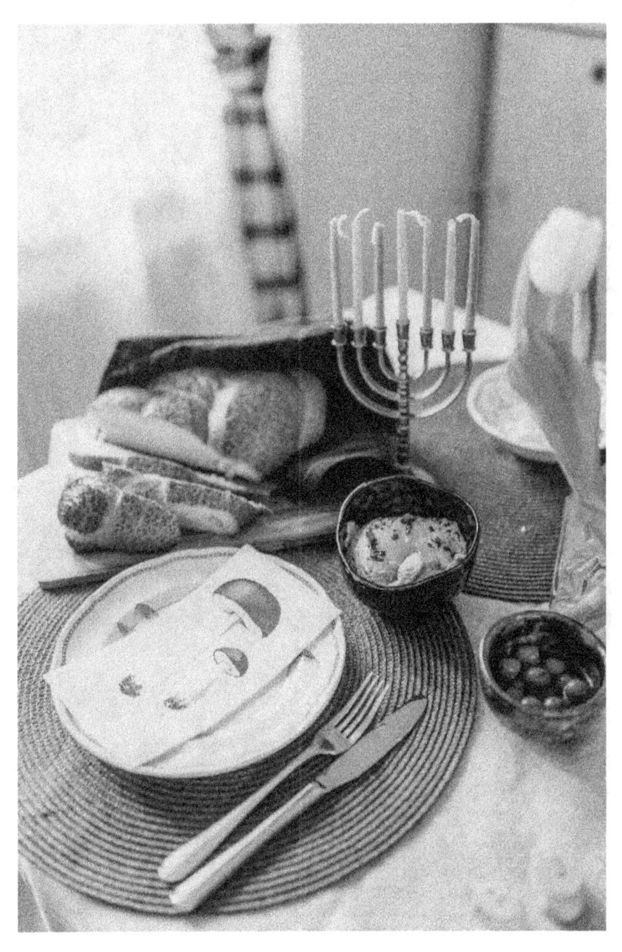

| GALVESTON COOKBOOK RECIPE

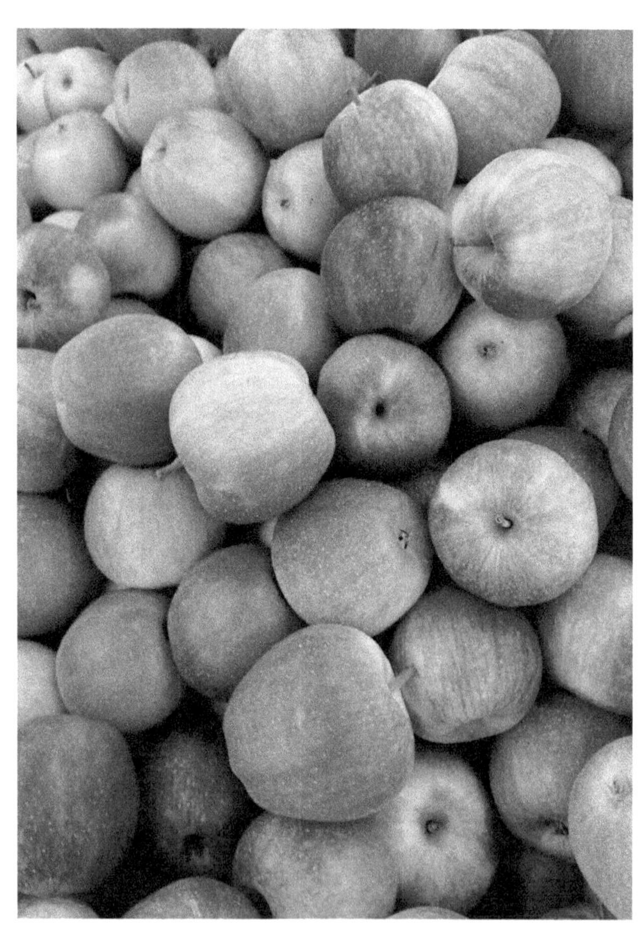

| GALVESTON COOKBOOK RECIPE

Chapter 4: Island-Inspired Beverages

Welcome to a tropical paradise within the pages of "The Galveston Cookbook." The fifth chapter is a delightful voyage through "Island-Inspired Beverages," which condenses the tastes of Galveston's coastal charm into elegant and delectable cocktails.

- ❖ **Serenity Cocktail:** Sunset Breeze Cocktail

  Consider the bright, golden hues of a sunset in Galveston reflected in a glass.

  The Sunset Breeze Cocktail takes you to the island's calm beaches with a relaxing blend of tropical juices, rum, and a touch of coconut cream. This chapter will show you how to create this cocktail, which has a taste of perfect calm and reflects the essence of Galveston's coastal magnificence.

- ❖ **Gulf Breeze Mocktail:** A Cooling Retreat

  The Gulf Breeze Mocktail is a delightful non-alcoholic solution for folks wanting a respite from alcohol. Consider a glass filled with sparkling water, citrus juices, and grenadine.

It's a mocktail as colorful and exhilarating as a swim in the Gulf. A portion supports you in making an alcohol-free delight ideal for persons of all ages.

❖ **Paloma Fresca:** Spicy and Fizzy

Our adventure continues with the Paloma Fresca, a spicy and effervescent beverage as vivid as Galveston. It's a drink that dances on your taste buds, prepared with tequila, grapefruit soda, and a touch of fresh lime.

In this section, you'll learn how to polish the Paloma Fresca, echoing the bright exuberance of Galveston's island culture.

❖ **A Taste of Paradise:** Tropical Fruit Punch

This chapter finishes with a taste of paradise—the Tropical Fruit Punch. Consider a pitcher full of tropical fruits, juices, and a dash of coconut water.

It's a punch as vivid and colorful as the island's greenery. You'll learn how to produce this beautiful masterpiece, a drink that brings the tastes of

Galveston's tropical refuge to your table, in this section.

Chapter 4 is a taste of island-inspired enjoyment, with each beverage reflecting Galveston's beachside splendor. By the end of this chapter, you'll not only have a range of refreshing cocktails at your disposal.

but also a strong grasp of the island's lively culture, where every drink embodies the laid-back elegance and tropical appeal that define Galveston's attitude.

Galveston's Signature Cocktails

Prepare to embark on a libation discovery journey as we delve into Chapter 4 of "The Galveston Cookbook" - "Galveston's Signature Cocktails.

" This chapter is a thrilling voyage into the realm of mixology, where the island's distinct flavors and coastal charm are translated into trademark beverages that embody Galveston's character.

The Signature Cocktail Experience at Island Elegance Imagine resting on a breezy waterfront patio, staring out at the gorgeous Gulf waters while sipping a freshly crafted drink.

This is the core of Galveston's Signature Cocktails—a terrific and delightful experience. In this phase, you'll learn the art of mixology and how to produce these one-of-a-kind cocktails inspired by the island's culture.

❖ **Sunset Breeze Cocktail:** A Serene Sip

The Sunset Breeze Cocktail is the first destination on our adventure. Consider the sun sinking over the horizon, illuminating the sky with warm, golden hues—the inspiration for this calming libation.

This cocktail combines the essence of a Galveston sunset in a glass, with a blend of tropical juices, a dash of rum, and a touch of coconut cream. Learn how to prepare this drink, a taste of pure calm that takes you to the island's quiet coasts.

❖ **Gulf Breeze Mocktail:** A Refreshing Oasis for People of All Ages

The Gulf Breeze Mocktail is a nice non-alcoholic alternative for folks who desire to avoid alcohol. Consider the wonderful sea air on your face as you sip sparkling water blended with citrus fruits and grenadine.

It's a mocktail as colorful and exhilarating as a swim in the Gulf. A portion supports you in making an alcohol-free delight ideal for persons of all ages.

❖ **Paloma Fresca:** A Spicy Dance for Your Palate

Our voyage continues with the Paloma Fresca, a peppery and effervescent beverage that embodies Galveston's vivacious nature.

It's a drink that dances on your taste buds, prepared with tequila, grapefruit soda, and a dash of fresh lime. During this phase, you'll improve the method of blending the Paloma Fresca, embodying the exuberant essence of Galveston's island culture.

❖ **Tropical Fruit Punch:** A Flavor of Paradise

This chapter finishes with a taste of tropical paradise—the Tropical Fruit Punch. Consider a pitcher full of tropical fruits, a symphony of juices, and a dash of coconut water.

It's a punch as vivid and colorful as the island's greenery. You'll learn how to produce this beautiful masterpiece, a drink that brings the tastes of Galveston's tropical refuge to your table, in this section.

The Signature Cocktails of Galveston are more than simply cocktails; they are expressions of the island's beauty and coastal charm. By the conclusion of this segment, you'll not only have a repertory of refreshing.

concoctions under your belt but also a greater connection to Galveston's culture, where every sip embodies the island's laid-back elegance and tropical charm. Cheers to Galveston's one-of-a-kind cocktail culture!

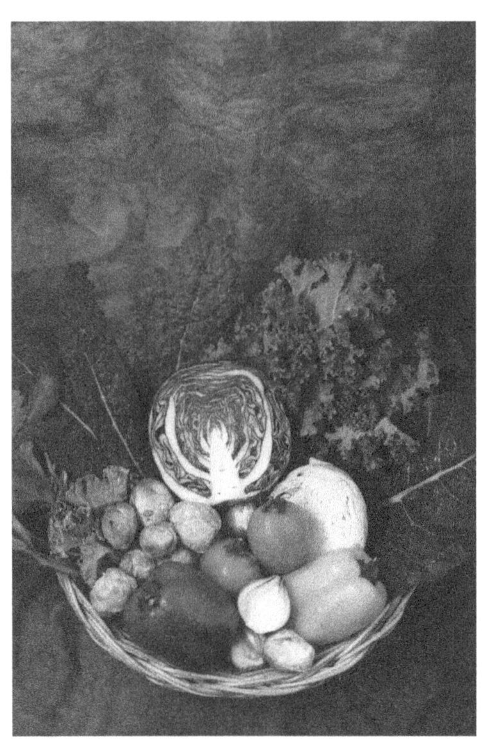

| GALVESTON COOKBOOK RECIPE

Tropical Fruit Smoothies

Prepare to be transported to a tropical paradise as we explore Chapter 4 of "The Galveston Cookbook" - "Tropical Fruit Smoothies." This is a tranquil sanctuary where the tastes of Galveston's lush surroundings and beachside grandeur are mixed into vivid and interesting cocktails.

- ❖ **Island Breeze Smoothie:** A Tropical Sip

  Imagine yourself standing on a pristine beach, feeling the cold wind on your skin and tasting the tastes of the tropics.

  This sensation is encapsulated by the Island Breeze Smoothie. It's created with fresh pineapple, and creamy coconut milk, with a tinge of tart citrus.

  In this episode, you'll discover how to create this smoothie, a drink that takes you to Galveston's tropical splendor with every sip.

- ❖ **Mango Tango Smoothie:** A Flavor Dance

The Mango Tango Smoothie is a colorful ballet of flavors that satisfies the senses. Consider luscious and aromatic mangoes paired with creamy Greek yogurt and a touch of honey.

This smoothie is a celebration of the blend of sweet and acidic ingredients. In this episode, you'll discover how to prepare the Mango Tango Smoothie, a dance on your taste senses that embodies the spirit of Galveston's tropical grandeur.

Creamy Bliss Coconut Paradise Smoothie

Our trip continues with the Coconut Paradise Smoothie, a creamy and delightful combination that tastes like pure happiness. Imagine a velvety blend of creamy coconut milk, succulent bananas, and a dash of vanilla This smoothie is like a drink of peace.

in the middle of the island's vivid grandeur In this part, you'll learn how to prepare the Coconut Paradise Smoothie, a creamy delicacy that comforts the spirit.

❖ **Sunset Serenade Smoothie:** A Sweet and Tangy

This chapter finishes with a sweet and tangy treat: the Sunset Serenade Smoothie.

Consider a lovely sunset over the Gulf reflected in a glass of exquisite peaches, sharp raspberries, and a dash of lime. It's a smoothie that plays a symphony of fruity notes on your taste senses.

This chapter will show you how to prepare the Sunset Serenade Smoothie, a drink that simulates the beautiful hues of a Galveston sunset.

The Tropical Fruit Smoothies in "The Galveston Cookbook" are more than simply drinks; they're a voyage through the island's natural beauty and bright surroundings.

By the conclusion of this part, you'll not only have a collection of delightful recipes but also a stronger connection to Galveston's green environs, where each sip represents the island's tropical charm and coastal calm. Cheers to the great taste!

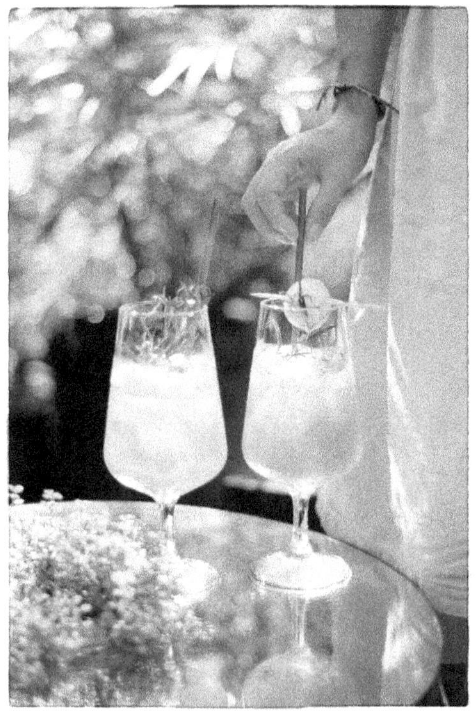

Fresh Sea Breeze Mocktail

As we explore Chapter 4 of "The Galveston Cookbook," "Fresh Sea Breeze Mocktail," we will enter a universe of seaside tranquillity and refreshing sips. This cocktail pays honor to Galveston's serene beauty by mixing the essence of the sea with the freshness of citrus.

❖ **The Sea's Embrace:** A Serenity Mocktail Imagine meandering around Galveston's sandy beaches, feeling the sea wind caress your skin.

This tranquil mood is conveyed by the Fresh Sea Breeze Mocktail. It's a wonderful combination of oceanic tastes, with the brightness of fresh citrus, the sharpness of cranberry juice, and the fizz of soda water.

You'll discover how to prepare this mocktail, a sip of beautiful coastal calm that transfers the sea to your glass, in this segment.

❖ **Fresh Citrus Symphony:** A Palate Dance

A symphony of fresh citrus is at the center of the Fresh Sea Breeze Mocktail. Consider the brightness of a lime slice, the zing of juicy oranges, and the acidity of cranberries.

These components blend in a faultless dance on your tongue, producing a symphony of tastes that is both refreshing and exhilarating. This course will show you how to precisely blend these citrus tones.

❖ **Soda Sparkle:** Elegance and Effervescence

The effervescence of this mocktail adds greatly to its attractiveness. Soda water adds a touch of refinement, generating small bubbles that pleasure your senses with each drink.

Learn how to master the art of effervescence to make your Fresh Sea Breeze Mocktail as delightful as a plunge in the Gulf waves.

❖ **A Coastal Toast:** A Sip of Tranquility in Galveston

The Fresh Sea Breeze Mocktail is more than simply a drink; it's a seaside salute to the peacefulness of Galveston's coastlines.

By the conclusion of this part, you'll not only have a refreshing mocktail recipe but also a better connection to the island's calm beauty, where every sip epitomizes.
the laid-back elegance and natural grandeur that characterize Galveston's attitude. Cheers to the flavor of the sea wind!

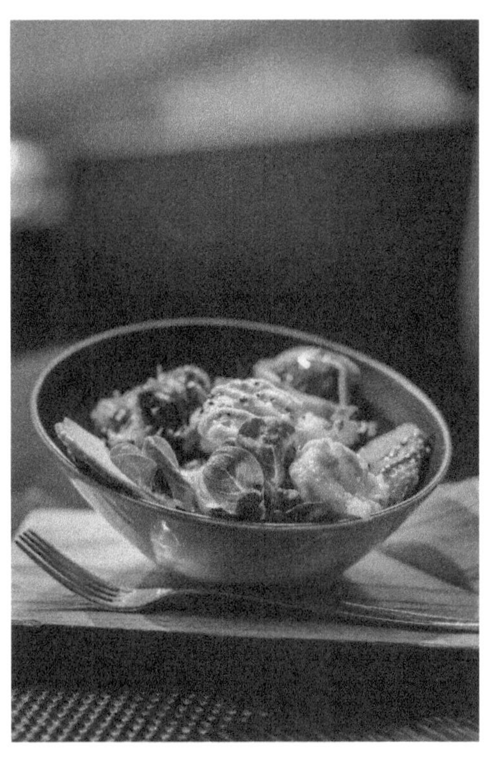

| GALVESTON COOKBOOK RECIPE

Chapter 5: Farm-to-Table Galveston

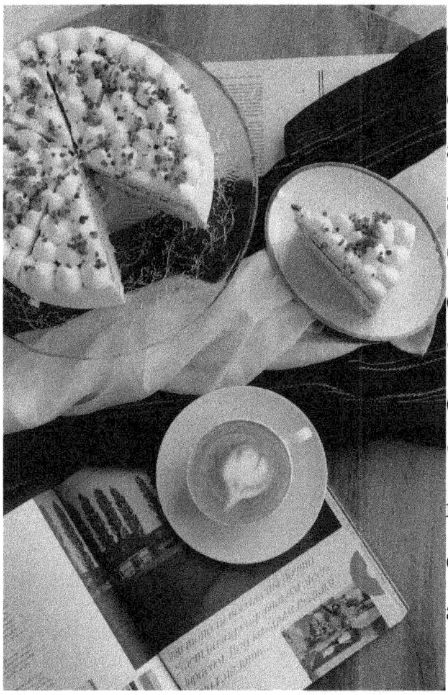

Prepare to travel on a culinary trip that celebrates the freshness and taste of locally sourced foods in Chapter 6 of "The Galveston Cookbook" - "Farm-to-Table Galveston." This chapter is a monument to the island's devotion to sustainable and excellent cuisine, with a focus on the richness of local farms and fisheries.

Fresh Farmers' Markets in Galveston: A Culinary Treasure Trove

In this episode, we explore Galveston's crowded Farmers' Markets, where we discover the island's gastronomic treasures. Picture booths packed with lovely fruits, fresh veggies, and artisan goods.

Learn the value of supporting local farmers and how to pick the freshest ingredients to take your cuisine to the next level.

❖ **Coastal Catch:** Galveston's Waters' Bounty

The Gulf of Mexico offers a plethora of seafood, and this part digs into the skill of selecting and cooking the freshest fish.

From juicy Gulf shrimp to delicate red snapper, you'll discover how to blend the tastes of the seas into your cuisine. Discover the secrets of picking fish, from detecting freshness to ecologically responsible alternatives.

❖ **Garden-to-Table:** Bringing Galveston Flavors to Life

As we study the Garden-to-Table idea, get your hands dirty in Galveston's gardens. Discover the island's vibrant communal gardens and how to cultivate your own herbs and veggies. Learn the significance of organic and sustainable ways of cultivating your ingredients, and learn how to infuse your dishes with the genuine flavor of Galveston's gardens.

❖ **Traditional Recipes:** A Taste of Local Delights

The food inspired by local products is at the center of Farm-to-Table Galveston. This section features a range of meals that pay respect to the island's culinary tradition. Each meal is a celebration of Galveston's farm-to-table ethos, from seafood gumbo packed with Gulf   pleasures

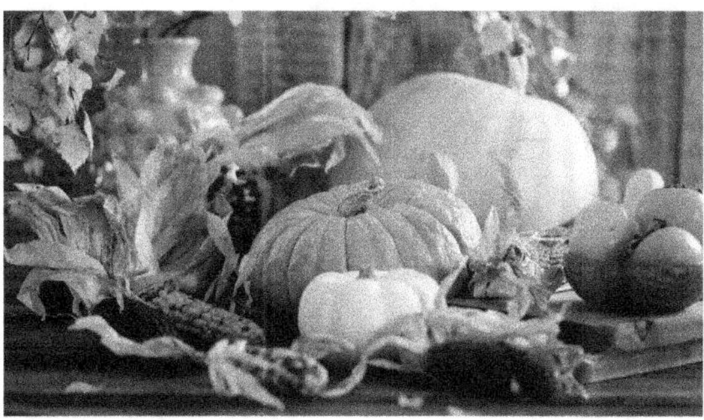

to fresh vegetable salads brimming with flavor.

A Culinary Legacy and the Joy of Sustainability

Sustainability is more than a slogan in Galveston; it is a way of life.

This section will inform you about the island's dedication to sustainable eating and how you may assist the environment while enjoying excellent meals. Discover the wonders of sustainability and its long-lasting influence on Galveston's culinary heritage.

Chapter 5 recognizes the island's devotion to quality, freshness, and the preservation of local customs by the end of this chapter, you'll not only have a better understanding of Farm-to-Table.

Galveston but also the knowledge and skills to create dishes that capture the essence of the island's commitment to sustainable and delicious dining—a cuisine that nourishes both the body and the soul while supporting local communities.

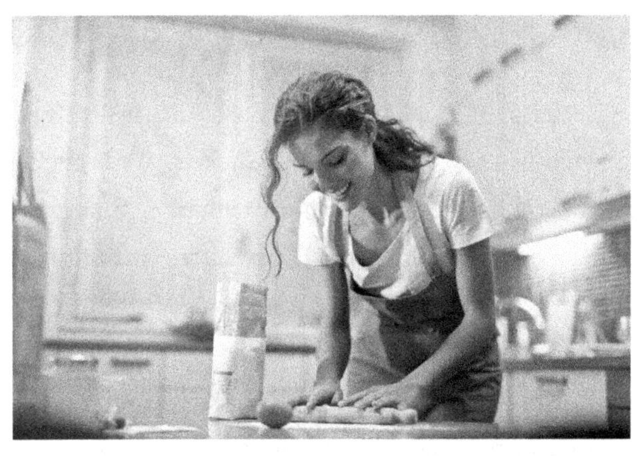

| GALVESTON COOKBOOK RECIPE

Exploring Local Farmers' Markets

In Chapter 5 of "The Galveston Cookbook," you'll visit the hectic world of Galveston's Farmers' Markets. We begin our trip into the core of the island's culinary culture here, stressing the complex tapestry of tastes and ingredients obtained from local farmers and craftsmen.

- ❖ **Farmers' Market Essence:** A Culinary Treasure Trove

  Consider meandering through open-air marketplaces draped with colorful canopies, a symphony of fragrances floating through the air.

  Galveston's Farmers' Markets are a gastronomic treasure trove, providing fresh, seasonal crops, artisan products, and a connection to the local community. In this part, you'll learn about the principles of Farmers' Markets and their relevance in sustaining Galveston's cuisines.

- ❖ **Supporting Local:** Farmers' Markets at Their Best

Farmers' markets are more than simply places to buy; they give a chance to support local farmers, craftsmen, and small businesses.

Learn about the importance of this connection and how your purchases directly affect the lives of people who grow the island's abundance. Discover the feeling of community and sustainability that permeates these busy markets.

❖ **Selecting Freshness:** A Local Ingredients Guide

Navigating Farmers' Markets is a talent in and of itself. This part will show you how to pick the freshest ingredients. You'll learn how to pick items that will improve your cuisine, from ripe, juicy tomatoes to aromatic herbs and excellent cheeses. Knowing the seasons and regional characteristics will help you to produce farm-to-table masterpieces.

A Culinary Adventure with Farmers' Market Treasures

Explore the varied choices at Galveston's Farmers' Markets. Imagine fresh tomatoes overflowing with flavor, honey acquired from local beehives, and homemade bread with a gorgeous crust.

In this area, you'll uncover the hidden gems just waiting to be unearthed and integrated into your culinary masterpieces.

❖ **A Taste of Galveston:** Recipes with a Fresh Twist

The dishes inspired by Farmers' Market findings constitute the center of this chapter. From farm-fresh salads to vivid fruit tarts, you'll have the chance to cook meals that celebrate Galveston's particular qualities. Each dinner is a celebration of the island's culinary culture, showcasing market preferences.

Exploring local farmers' markets is a cultural experience that enhances your relationship with the community, encourages sustainability, and enables you to sample the essence of Galveston's cuisines.

By the conclusion of this part, you'll not only have a greater appreciation for the island's Farmers' Markets but also the knowledge and motivation to integrate the richness of local ingredients into your culinary creations—a cuisine that actually symbolizes Galveston's farm-to-table philosophy.

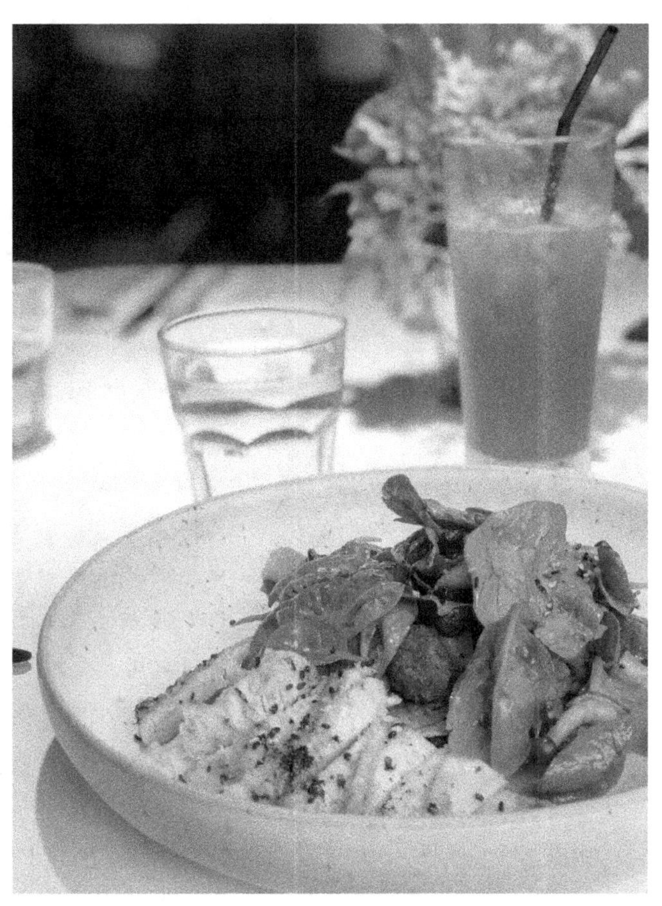

GALVESTON COOKBOOK RECIPE

Farm-Fresh Vegetable Medley

Prepare to be amazed by the brilliant colors and tastes in Chapter 5 of "The Galveston Cookbook" as we explore the delightful "Farm-Fresh Vegetable Medley.

" In this area, we celebrate the abundance of Galveston's local farms, where each product is a piece of beauty in its own right.

- ❖ **Nature's Masterpiece:** The Vegetable Palette

    Consider a palette of fresh veggies, each one a brushstroke of bright color and unique taste. The Farm-Fresh Vegetable Medley is a culinary canvas that mixes the greatest crops of the season.

    Consider heirloom tomatoes, crisp bell peppers, delicate zucchini, and earthy carrots from your local producers. In this part, you'll learn how to blend different veggies to produce a medley that's not only aesthetically stunning but also a symphony of flavors and feelings.

A Tribute to Local Farms: The Freshest Ingredients

This meal is devoted to local farms—the unsung heroes that produce the island's tastes. Learn about the farmers and their dedication to adopting sustainable and organic practices to produce the freshest meals.

Discover the satisfaction of knowing precisely where your veggies originate from and how they've been nurtured from seed to harvest.

The Art of Preparation in Farm-to-Table Magic

Making a Farm-Fresh Vegetable Medley is about more than just the ingredients; it's also about the art of preparation.

In this course, you'll learn how to accentuate the intrinsic characteristics of each vegetable by slicing, chopping, and roasting it. To guarantee that your combination is a culinary masterpiece, understand the value of time and seasoning.

❖ **The Finished Dish:** A Symphony of Tastes and Textures

The simplicity of the Farm-Fresh Vegetable Medley is its beauty. Consider a supper of roasted veggies drizzled with olive oil and sprinkled with sea salt.

Each mouthful is a delicious combination of flavors and textures—crispy, delicate, sweet, and salty. In this step, you'll go through the final presentation to ensure that your medley is not only tasty but also aesthetically stunning.

A Culinary Journey Celebrating Galveston Flavors

The Farm-Fresh Vegetable Medley is more than simply a dinner; it's a culinary excursion through the tastes of Galveston's local farms. By the conclusion of this segment, you'll have not just a great dinner but also a better awareness of the artistry of farm-to-table cooking.

You'll have the expertise and drive to construct meals that showcase the essence of local produce—a cuisine that actually represents Galveston's dedication tosustainability and appreciation for nature's abundance.

Sustainable Seafood Stew

Prepare to enjoy the ambiance of Galveston's coastal appeal as we dig into Chapter 5 of "The Galveston Cookbook" - "Sustainable Seafood Stew.

" This supper is a celebration of the Gulf's wealth, made with a dedication to sustainability and a love of the ocean's bounty.

Nature's Bounty: A Symphony of Seafood

Consider a saucepan cooking with a symphony of Gulf of Mexico flavors.

Sustainable Seafood Stew is a gastronomic voyage through the ocean's treasures, featuring plump Gulf shrimp, soft red snapper, sweet blue crab, and more.

Each component is carefully chosen to guarantee its long-term survival while also protecting the delicate balance of marine ecosystems.

In this part, you'll learn how to combine these seafood pearls into a healthy and environmentally beneficial stew.

❖ **Honoring the Ocean:** The Legacy of Sustainability

At the core of this approach is a dedication to sustainability—the desire to maintain the ocean and its delicate ecosystems. Discover how sustainable seafood methods aid in the long-term health of marine life.

Recognize the significance of responsible fishing and procurement, ensuring that the seafood on your plate is the outcome of ethical and ecologically beneficial efforts.

- ❖ **Creating the Perfect Stew:** A Flavor Symphony

  Creating a Sustainable Seafood Stew is a culinary undertaking that takes accuracy and expertise.

  In this part, you'll learn how to simmer, season, and layer flavors to produce a rich, fragrant, and thoroughly enjoyable stew. Each taste is an invitation to appreciate the ocean's richness, from the first waft of simmering soup to the last sip.

- ❖ **A Feast for the Senses:** A Celebration of Galveston's Waters

  Consider a warm dish of Sustainable Seafood Stew—a sensory feast. The perfume of herbs and spices mingles with the smell of the sea, and the colors of the Gulf's abundance dance in the thick soup.

Each mouthful is a flavor explosion, a taste of Galveston's coastal history that takes you to the island's coastlines.

❖ **Embracing the Gifts of the Gulf:** A Culinary Legacy

Sustainable Seafood Stew is more than simply a meal; it's a culinary legacy that commemorates the Gulf's riches and the dedication to conserving them for future generations.

By the conclusion of this part, you'll not only have a beautiful dinner but also a better awareness of sustainable eating and the value of ethical choices in culinary endeavors—a cuisine that is both a celebration of taste and an homage to the ocean's everlasting beauty.

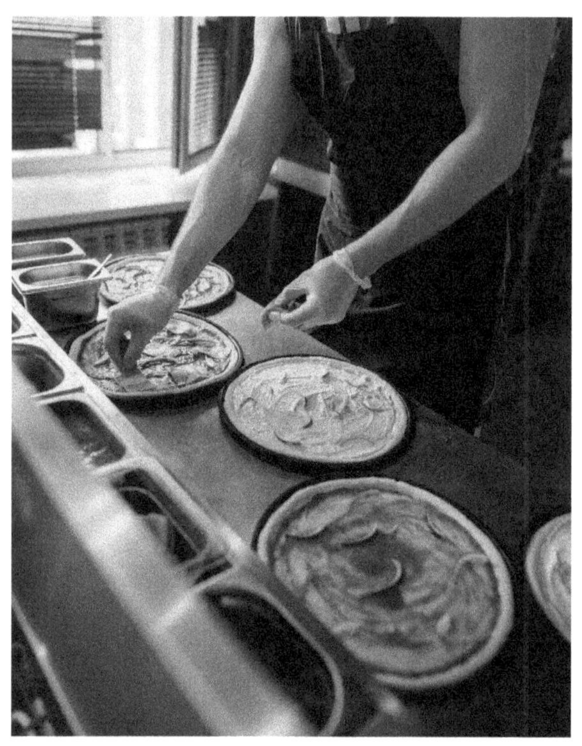

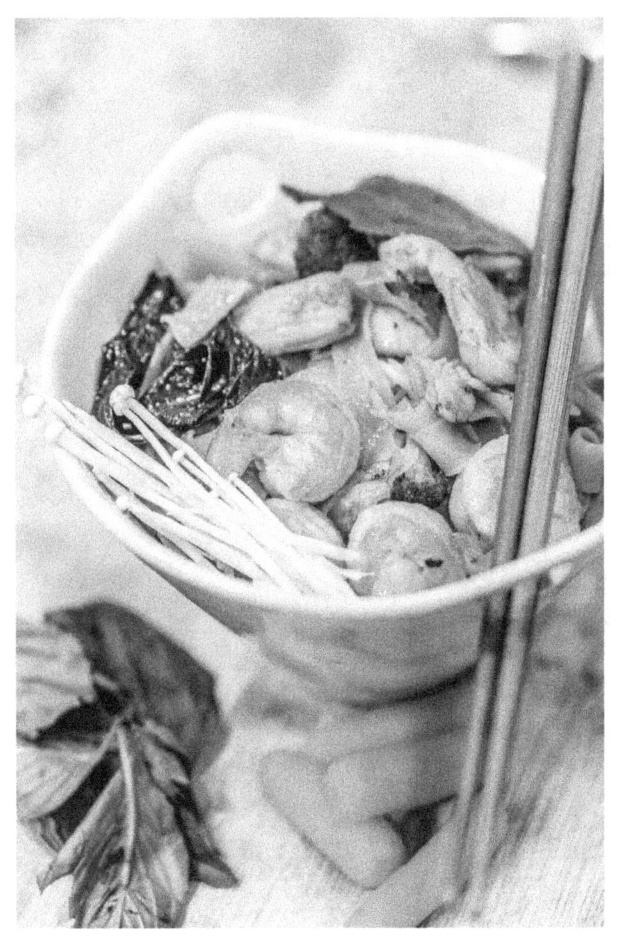

| GALVESTON COOKBOOK RECIPE

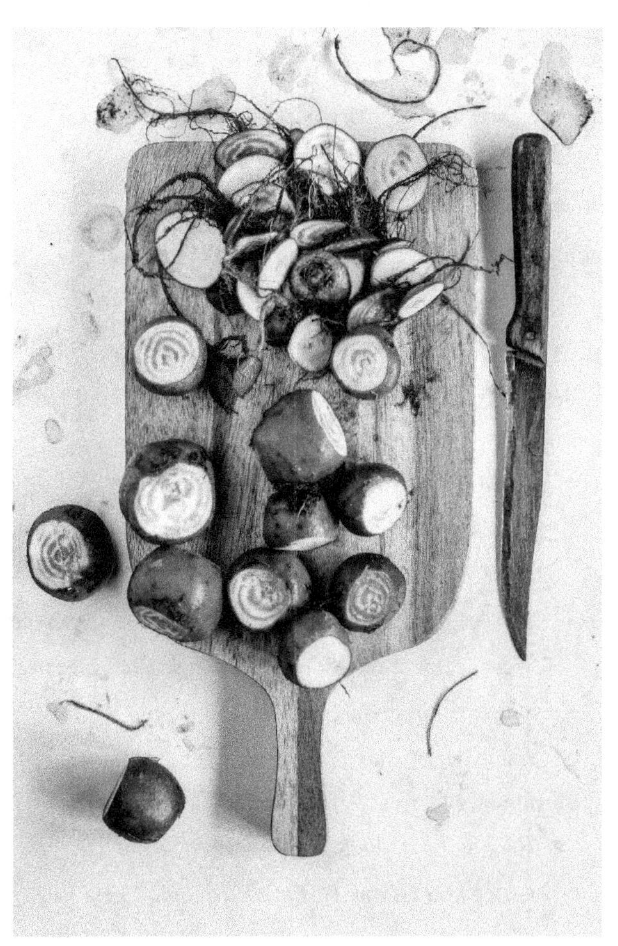

| GALVESTON COOKBOOK RECIPE

Chapter 6: Sweet Treats of Galveston

Indulge your sweet craving as we explore Chapter 6 of "The Galveston Cookbook" - "Sweet Treats of Galveston." This chapter is a lovely tour through the island's confectionary treats, with each mouthful a celebration of Galveston's dessert culture.

- ❖ **Gulf Coast Pralines:** Southern Elegance

  In this episode, we begin our sweet adventure with Gulf Coast Pralines, a traditional Southern delight that is as elegant as it is wonderful. Consider creamy, sweet confections topped with roasted pecans—a symphony of textures and tastes.

  You'll learn how to create delightful pralines, a bite-sized treat that reflects the warmth and friendliness of the South.

- ❖ **Galveston Island Taffy:** A Nostalgic Coast Bite

Galveston Island Taffy is more than just candy; it's a taste of nostalgia, bringing you to seaside boardwalks and salty sea breezes. In this episode, you'll learn how to prepare this chewy, delightful dessert.

Learn how to pull, twist, and mold taffy into wonderful delicacies that reflect the spirit of Galveston's coastal magnificence.

❖ **Key Lime Pie:** A Tart Slice of Paradise

Key Lime Pie is a taste of tropical paradise that mirrors the flavors of Galveston's oceanfront. Consider a buttery graham cracker crust topped with a cloud of whipped cream and filled with a creamy, tangy key lime filling.

In this segment, you'll learn how to prepare this renowned dessert, a taste of the Gulf's spicy appeal that takes you to sun-soaked coasts.

❖ **A Southern Classic:** Sweet Potato Pecan Pie

Sweet Potato Pecan Pie is a popular Southern dish that mixes the earthy sweetness of sweet potatoes with the rich, nutty taste of pecans. This chapter will

show you how to prepare this comfortable pie, a treat
that relates to the tastes and traditions of the South.

❖ **Ice Cream Dreams:** Flavors of Galveston

Ice cream is a universal delight, and we display
Galveston's distinct ice cream culture in this area.
Learn how to create smooth, creamy ice cream filled
with tropical tastes.

Whether it's tropical fruit sorbets or rich chocolate
pleasures, you'll be able to produce frozen sweets that
please the taste senses.

Chapter 6 is a delectable symphony, with each dessert
paying honor to Galveston's culinary tradition.

By the conclusion of this chapter, you'll not only have a
wonderful recipe collection, but also a better connection to the
island's dessert culture, where every taste symbolizes the joy
of indulgence and the celebration of life's sweet moments.

Key Lime Pie with Graham Cracker Crust

In Chapter 6 of "The Galveston Cookbook," we travel on a pleasant voyage into the world of Key Lime Pie with Graham Cracker Crust—a tropical piece of heaven that embodies the spirit of Galveston's beach charm.

- ❖ **Tropical Allure:** Key Lime Pie's Essence

  As you consume a piece of Key Lime Pie, imagine the taste of sunlight and sea on your lips. This dessert reflects the spirit of Galveston's tropical enchantment. At its center is a wonderful, velvety filling prepared with the juice of small, sour key limes—a zesty, lively taste that's beautifully matched with sweetness.

  This section leads you through the process of manufacturing this legendary delicacy, where each mouthful is a voyage for your taste sensations.

  Butter-Kissed Graham Cracker Crust

  The Graham Cracker Crust is the pie's base, concealed below the silky lime filling. Consider a buttery, golden crust that cracks at the touch of a fork, offering a delightful contrast to the acidic lime interior.

In this portion, you'll learn how to prepare this delicious and crumbly crust, a foundation that's more than merely a vessel but a key component of the pie's complete experience.

❖ **Achieving the Perfect Tartness:** A Balancing Act
Key Lime Pie is a precise combination of sweet and sour. Learn how to balance tastes by ensuring that the acidity of the key lime filling is precisely balanced by the sweetness of condensed milk and sugar.
Recognize the significance of utilizing fresh key limes, which offer a particular zest to the pie.

❖ **Aesthetic Elegance:** Whipped Cream Garnish
The presentation of Key Lime Pie is crucial to its beauty. Consider a slice topped with a cloud of freshly whipped cream—light, wonderful, and a great accompaniment to the hot filling.

Learn how to garnish with whipped cream to produce an aesthetic elegance that is as pleasing to the eyes as it is to the mouth.

❖ **A Slice of Paradise:** Tropical Indulgence

Key Lime Pie with Graham Cracker Crust is more than just dessert; it's a bit of tropical paradise on a plate, a taste of Galveston's beachfront grandeur.

By the conclusion of this section, you'll not only have a delectable recipe, but also a clearer grasp of the island's dessert culture, where every flavor symbolizes the colorful spirit of Galveston's sun-soaked shores—a dessert that's more than just a pleasure, but a culinary vacation to paradise.

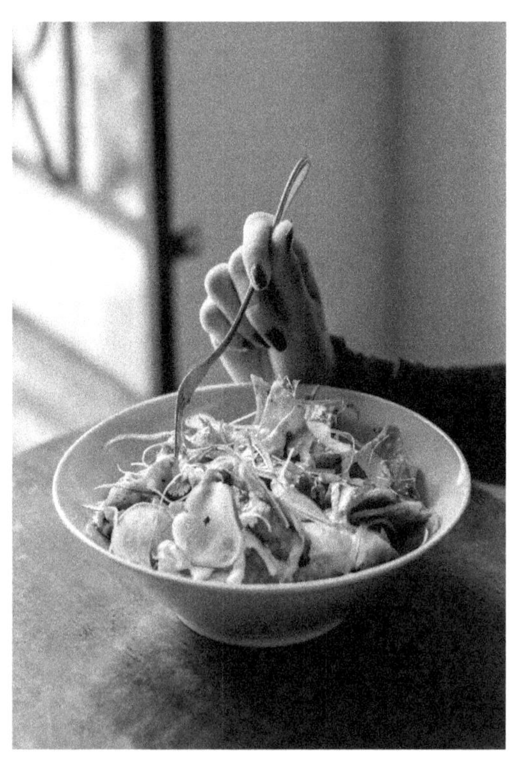

Sweet Southern Elegance Pecan Pralines me

Enter a land of sweet southern elegance in Chapter 6 of "The Galveston Cookbook" as we explore the delicious kingdom of Pecan Pralines. These delights are a testament to Galveston's warm hospitality and the rich tastes of the South.

- ❖ **A Symphony of Sweetness:** Unveiling Pecan Pralines

  Consider a dessert that mixes sweet, creamy caramel with the buttery richness of almonds. Pecan Pralines are a delightful symphony that takes you to a realm of southern charm.

  In this part, you'll learn how to create these beautiful delights, where each mouthful is a taste of Galveston's warm embrace.

- ❖ **Pecans:** The Praline's Heart

  The fundamental components of Pecan Pralines are pecans, which are famed for their buttery taste and exquisite crunch.

Learn how to pick the best nuts and roast them to perfection, boosting their nutty taste and giving depth to the pralines.

- ❖ **The Caramelization Magic:** Creating Praline Perfection

Making Pecan Pralines is a delightful caramelization experience. In this course, you'll learn how to boil sugar and cream to produce a wonderful caramel foundation. Learn how to acquire the perfect consistency and color to fill each praline with a velvety, melt-in-your-mouth sensation.

Manufactured Delights: Shaping and Setting

Making Pecan Pralines is an artistic procedure that enables you to generate unique masterpieces.

Learn how to spoon out dollops of caramel and pecans onto parchment paper so they can cool and solidify into wonderful confections.

The technique is not merely tasty, but also tactile, connecting you to the art of making sweet southern beauty.

- ❖ **A Bite of Tradition:** A Taste of Southern Heritage

Pecan Pralines are more than simply sweets; they're a taste of southern tradition, a flavor of Galveston's welcoming attitude.

By the conclusion of this segment, you'll not only have a tasty supper but also a deeper knowledge of Southern culinary conventions. Each Pecan Praline highlights the region's rich tastes and traditions, encouraging you to feel the essence of southern elegance with each mouthful.

Galveston Gulf Coast Taffy

Chapter 6 of "The Galveston Cookbook" brings you to a coastal boardwalk where the air is filled with the exquisite aroma of Galveston Gulf Coast Taffy—a lovely delicacy that evokes the nostalgia of seaside vacations and the majesty of the Gulf.

A Taste of Coastal Nostalgia: The Unveiling of Galveston Gulf Coast Taffy

Close your eyes and envision the sounds of seagulls, the feel of sand on your feet, and the taste of salt in the air.

Galveston Gulf Coast Taffy is a bite-sized slice of coastal nostalgia, conjuring recollections of beach boardwalks and carefree days by the ocean.

In this part, you'll learn how to prepare this chewy, aromatic treat that symbolizes Galveston's seaside charm.

- ❖ **The Taffy-Making Tradition:** A Seaside Adventure Creating Gulf Coast Taffy is a coastal ritual that stretches back centuries. Consider a taffy puller in action, masterfully stretching and folding the candy to produce its trademark chewiness.

Learn the art of manufacturing taffy and how to acquire the precise texture that makes each bite a joy.

❖ **Coast Flavors:** Creating Taffy Varieties

Gulf Coast Taffy is offered in a range of flavors, ranging from basic vanilla and chocolate to tropical coconut and fruity pleasures.

In this course, you'll learn how to flavor and color taffy, enabling you to make a range of delicacies that represent the lively coastal culture.

❖ **Aromatic Memories:** Homemade Taffy

Creating the Gulf Coast manufacturing taffy at home is about more than simply manufacturing sweets; it's about building aromatic memories. In this part, you'll discover how to correctly heat sugar and corn syrup, infusing the taffy with a lovely perfume that will fill your kitchen and your senses.

Shaping and Cutting Taffy Twists

Gulf Coast Taffy shape and cutting is a hands-on practice that enables you to be creative.

Learn how to construct ropes out of taffy, twist them into inventive forms, and cut them into bite-sized pieces.

The process is more than simply culinary; it's an artistic journey that ties you to the skill of crafting wonderful beach memories.

A Coastal Connection: Savoring the Flavor of Galveston

Gulf Coast Taffy is more than just candy; it's a bite-sized piece of coastal connection—a taste of Galveston's lively culture and seaside attraction.

By the conclusion of this portion, you'll not only have a fantastic lunch but also a deeper knowledge of coastal culinary traditions.

Every chewy mouthful of taffy embodies the nostalgia and beauty of Galveston's Gulf Coast, urging you to enjoy the spirit of seaside holidays.

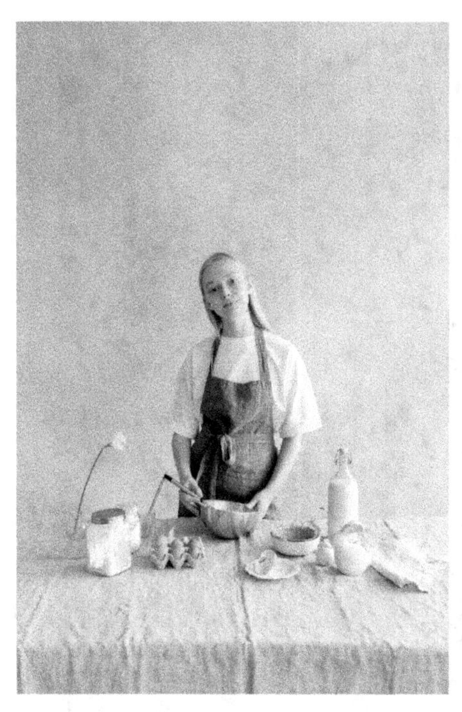

| GALVESTON COOKBOOK RECIPE

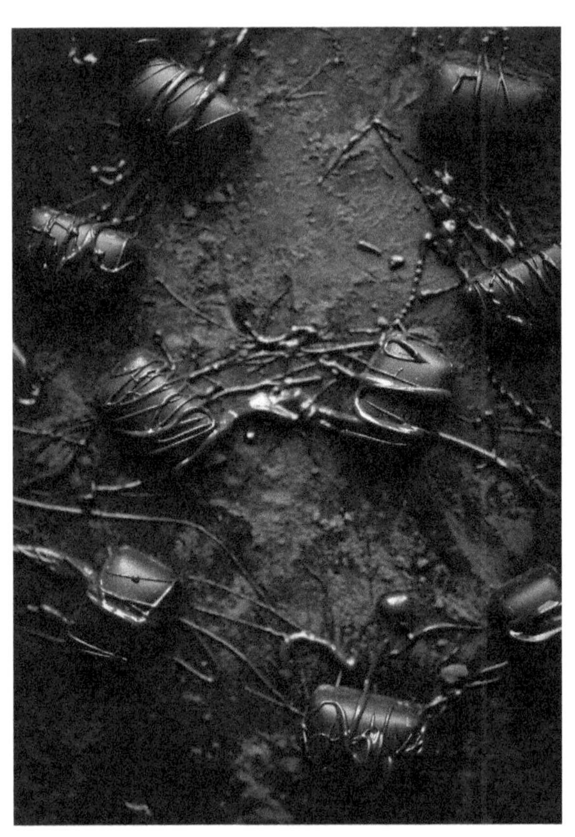

| GALVESTON COOKBOOK RECIPE

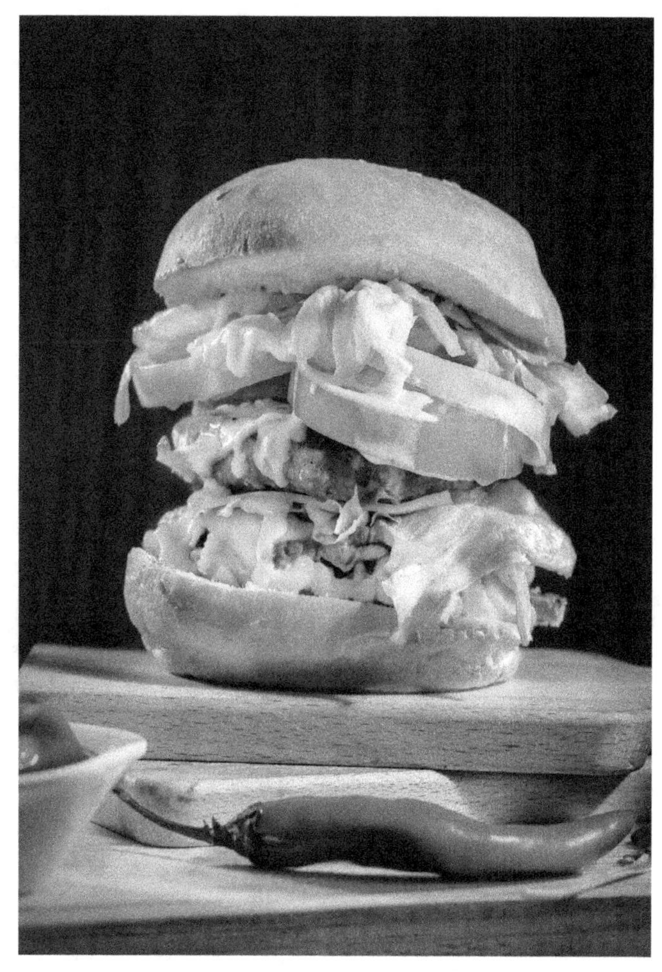

| GALVESTON COOKBOOK RECIPE

Chapter 7: Outdoor Cooking and Barbecue

Welcome to a blistering tour through "The Galveston Cookbook" Chapter 7 - "Outdoor Cooking and Barbecue." This chapter goes into Galveston's infatuation with open-air grilling, smokey tastes, and the thrill of cooking and eating beneath the Texas sun.

- ❖ **Gulf Coast Barbecue:** A Smoky Symphony

  In this episode, we go into the domain of Gulf Coast BBQ, a smokey symphony of smells that is an important component of Galveston's culinary culture. Consider delicate ribs, briskets, and sausages slow-cooked to perfection, each mouthful flavored with the taste of wood smoke.

  You'll learn about the smoking technique, wood selection, and the secrets of delicate, tasty Texas barbecue.

- ❖ **Beachside Grilling:** The Seafood Grillmasters

Beachfront grilling is an art form on Galveston's coastlines. This part will show you how to prepare fish to perfection.

From fresh Gulf shrimp to flaky snapper fillets, you'll learn how to employ open flames to accentuate the natural flavors of seafood, resulting in meals that embody the Gulf's richness.

❖ **Campfire Cooking:** Starry Nights

Consider sitting around a campfire beneath a starry Texas sky, with the fragrance of smokey deliciousness floating through the air. Campfire cooking is a beloved tradition, and in this part, you'll learn how to create wonderful meals in the great outdoors.

From foil-package meals to cast-iron pan sweets, you'll learn the delights of campfire cooking.

❖ **Tex-Mex BBQ Fiesta:** Spicy Southwest Flavors

Galveston's barbecue culture blends ingredients such as Tex-Mex with smokey barbecue.

This section will immerse you in the world of Tex-Mex BBQ, where spices, salsas, and robust tastes take center stage. Learn how to cook wonderful BBQ foods with a fiery southwestern taste that is distinctly Galveston.

❖ **Picnic Perfection:** Outdoor Dining

fresco eating is a way of life in Galveston, and this section will show you how to cook picnic-worthy dishes.

Consider a variety of sandwiches, salads, and cool drinks served in the great outdoors. Discover packing suggestions, portable meals, and how to construct magnificent picnics that embody the heart of Galveston's outdoor eating culture.

Chapter is a fiery ode to the tastes of outdoor cooking and barbecue, with each meal a celebration of Galveston's love of open-air eating and smoky, grilled delectability.

By the end of this chapter, you'll not only have a collection of delectable recipes, but also a stronger connection to the island's outdoor culinary culture—a cuisine that's about more than just the food, but also the experience of cooking and dining in the great outdoors, surrounded by the natural beauty of Galveston's landscapes

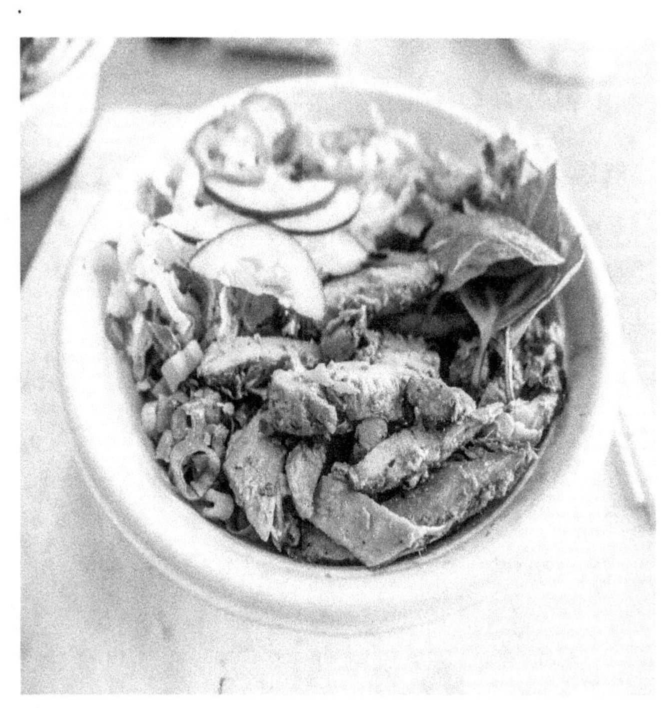

| GALVESTON COOKBOOK RECIPE

Galveston Grilled Gulf Shrimp Skewers

In Chapter 7 of "The Galveston Cookbook," we travel on a lovely voyage through the smoky, grilled tastes of Galveston with "Galveston Grilled Gulf Shrimp Skewers." These skewers are an homage to the Gulf's abundance and the art of outdoor grilling, which is firmly embedded in the island's heritage.

- ❖ **Galveston's Shrimp Delight:** The Gulf's Bounty on a Skewer

  Consider plump Gulf shrimp caressed by the flames of an open grill, their tastes accentuated by the smokiness of the grill.

  The Galveston Grilled Gulf Shrimp Skewers are a culinary marvel that embodies the essence of the Gulf's riches.

This part will show you how to grill shrimp to perfection so that each mouthful has a flavor of Galveston's beachside magnificence.

❖ **A Gulf Coast Tradition:** Choosing the Freshest Shrimp

The selection of components is vital to this cuisine. Learn how to pick the freshest Gulf shrimp, ensuring that they are tasty, sweet, and full of flavor.

Understand the significance of sustainable choices and how supporting local fisheries helps to maintain the Gulf's natural beauty.

Flavor Infusion Marination Magic

It's all about flavor infusion when it comes to producing delectable Galveston Grilled Gulf Shrimp Skewers.

| GALVESTON COOKBOOK RECIPE

In this segment, you'll learn how to marinade shrimp using a combination of spices, herbs, and a touch of citrus to enhance their natural taste.

Recognize the significance of marination time in creating the ideal balance of taste.

❖ **Skewer Artistry:** Skewer Assembly

Skewer construction is a creative method that lets you experiment with various colors and textures.

Consider huge prawns strung on skewers with bright veggies like bell peppers and onions. Learn how to skewer, making sure that each ingredient is appropriately positioned for uniform cooking and an aesthetically beautiful look.

❖ **Grillmaster Techniques:** The Perfect Grill

Grilling Galveston Grilled Gulf Shrimp Skewers needs some grillmaster talents. This part will delve into the art of grilling, from preheating the grill to creating the appropriate grill marks and smokey tastes.

Understand the timing for precisely cooked shrimp that are soft and imbued with grill flavor.

Savoring the Skewers at a Gulf Coast Feast Galveston Grilled Gulf Shrimp Skewers are a Gulf Coast feast in and of themselves.

By the conclusion of this segment, you'll not only have a great lunch but also a deeper connection to the island's enjoyment of outdoor cooking and the exhilaration of eating beneath the Texas sun.

Each skewer epitomizes the smoky, grilled delectability that distinguishes Galveston's culinary tradition, encouraging you to experience the essence of coastal charm with each exquisite mouthful.

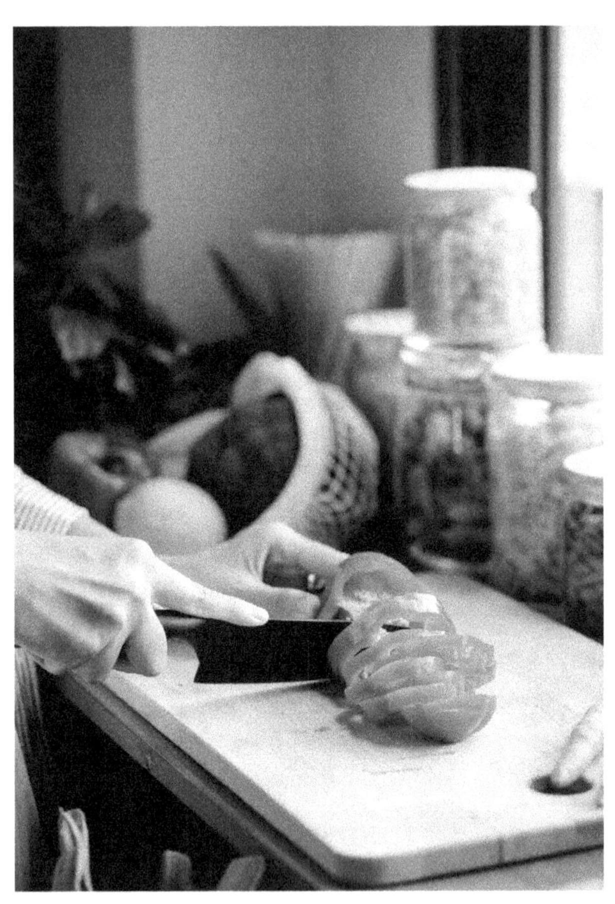

GALVESTON COOKBOOK RECIPE

Smoked Brisket with Homemade BBQ Sauce

With "Smoked Brisket with Homemade BBQ Sauce," we reach the world of exquisite, slow-smoked perfection in Chapter 8.2 of "The Galveston Cookbook.

" This is a genuine Texan favorite, and we'll look at how to obtain the delicate, smoky taste that marks Galveston's love for barbecue.

Galveston's BBQ Tradition: The Art of Smoked Brisket

Consider a huge brisket, nicely seasoned, gently cooking over a wood-fired pit. Smoked Brisket with Homemade BBQ Sauce is a culinary masterpiece that reflects Galveston's BBQ culture.

In this part, you'll learn about the art of smoking, how to pick the finest wood and the processes that result in delicate, tasty brisket.

How to Choose the Perfect Brisket: A BBQ Foundation

The choice of meat is vital to this dish. Learn how to pick the ideal brisket, one that's well-marbled and has just the proper proportion of fat to meat. Recognize the significance of trimming and seasoning so that every mouthful is a beautiful, smokey joy.

Slow and Low Smoking Magic

Getting the proper smokey taste requires time and precision. In this part, you'll learn about slow and low smoking, which enables the brisket to absorb the flavor of the wood while keeping its juiciness.

Learn about temperature control, smoke management, and the value of time in crafting melt-in-your-mouth tender brisket.

❖ **Homemade BBQ Sauce:** Flavor Booster

A nice BBQ sauce enhances any brisket. Learn how to create homemade BBQ sauce, which has an acidic, sweet, and smokey fragrance that lifts the brisket to new heights.

Understand the relevance of components such as ketchup, vinegar, brown sugar, and spices in attaining the appropriate taste balance.

❖ **The Finishing Touch:** Sauce Application
Applying BBQ sauce is an art form that completes your smoked brisket. In this part, you'll learn about basting, glazing, and offering sauce on the side to permit each client to personalize their brisket experience.

❖ **A Texas Barbecue Feast:** Brisket Savoring
The Smoked Brisket with Homemade BBQ Sauce is more than just a meal; it's a Texas barbecue feast.
By the conclusion of this portion, you'll not only have a tasty meal but also a stronger connection to the island's excitement for outdoor cooking and grilling.

Every delectable bite encapsulates the smoky,

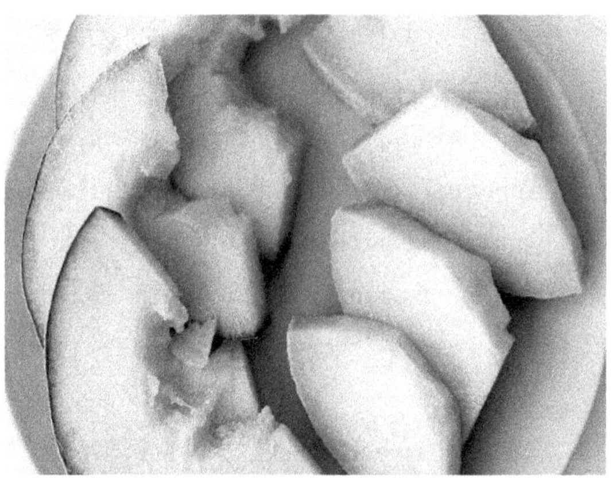

delicate sweetness that distinguishes Galveston's culinary tradition, letting you taste the essence of slow-smoked greatness.

Campfire Dutch Oven Cooking

In Chapter 7 of "The Galveston Cookbook," we continue on an adventurous excursion into the realm of Campfire Dutch Oven Cooking. This location invites you to explore the great outdoors, where campfires crackle and the fragrance of smokey goodness fills the air.

❖ **Galveston's Outdoor Tradition:** The Allure of Campfire Cooking

Consider yourself surrounded by nature's magnificence, with a bonfire creating a warm, flickering warmth.

Campfire Dutch Oven Cooking is a culinary experience profoundly steeped in Galveston's outdoor tradition. In this part, you'll experience the joy of creating wonderful meals in the outdoors, where each dish is imbued with natural tastes.

- ❖ **A Campfire Essential:** The Versatile Dutch Oven

    The Dutch oven is at the foundation of campfire cooking—a flexible and sturdy piece of equipment suited for outdoor culinary trips. Discover the numerous varieties of Dutch ovens, how to season and care for them, and why they're the favored option for campfire cooking.

- ❖ **Campfire Cuisine:** Recipes for Cooking Under the Stars

    Dutch Oven on the Campfire Cooking is a celebration of culinary ability as well as nourishment.

    In this area, you'll discover everything from substantial stews and savory casseroles to sweet cobblers and baked treats.

    Learn how to cook over an open flame, modify temperatures, and utilize coals to prepare wonderful campfire feasts.

- ❖ **Dutch Oven Desserts:** Wilderness Sweet Delights

    Dutch ovens are also fantastic for preparing exquisite treats. Consider warm, gooey cobblers and rich chocolate cakes cooked to perfection in the wide outdoors.

Discover the art of Dutch oven baking and how to produce delightful sweets that replicate the warmth of a campfire.

❖ **Campfire Essentials:** Fire Management and Safety

Cooking over a campfire involves particular abilities, such as fire control and safety. In this lesson, you'll learn how to create and maintain a campfire while keeping it safe for cooking. Recognize the significance of fire safety and authorized procedures of cooking in natural locations.

❖ **A Taste of the Wilderness:** Campfire Recipes

Campfire Dutch Oven Cooking is more than simply a meal; it's an engaging activity that links you to the beauty of nature.

By the conclusion of this part, you'll not only have a beautiful menu to pick from but also a stronger connection to the island's enjoyment of outdoor sports and the pleasure of dining under the stars.

Every exquisite taste exudes the smokey, rustic richness that distinguishes Galveston's campfire culture.

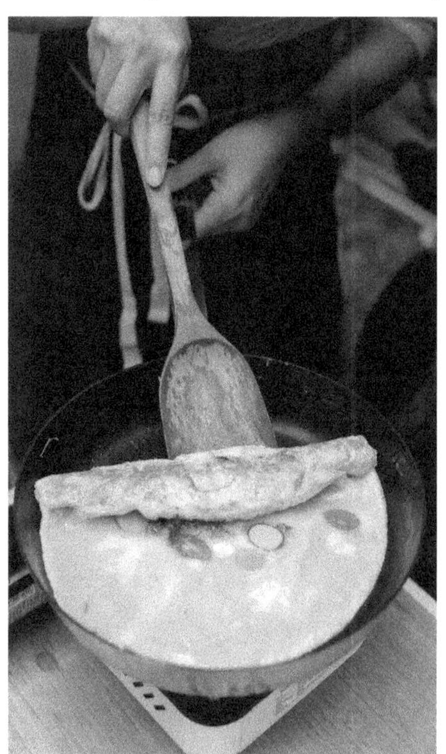

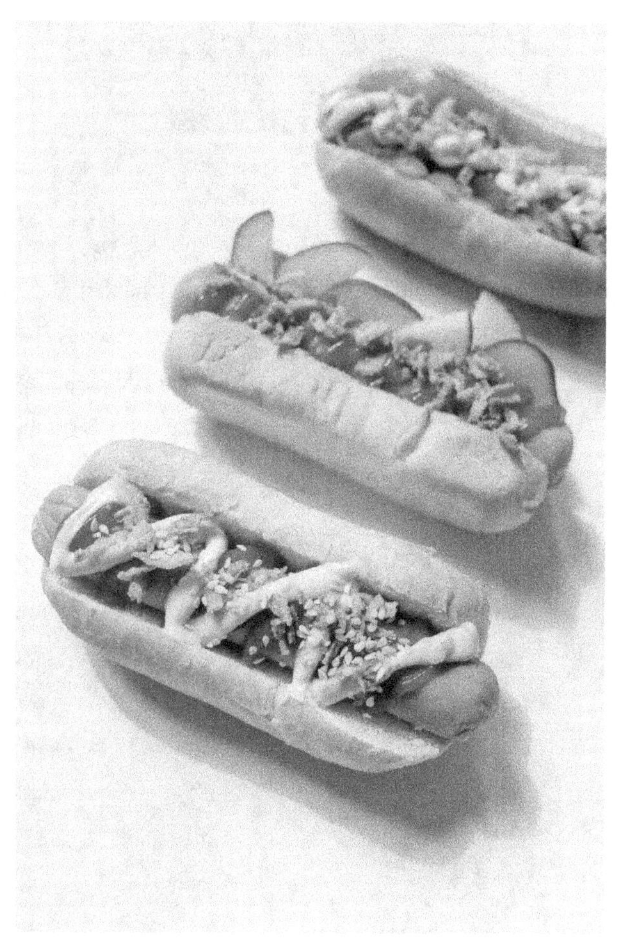

GALVESTON COOKBOOK RECIPE

Chapter 8: International Flavors in Galveston

In Chapter 8 of "The Galveston Cookbook," we take a culinary voyage throughout the world, studying the varied and

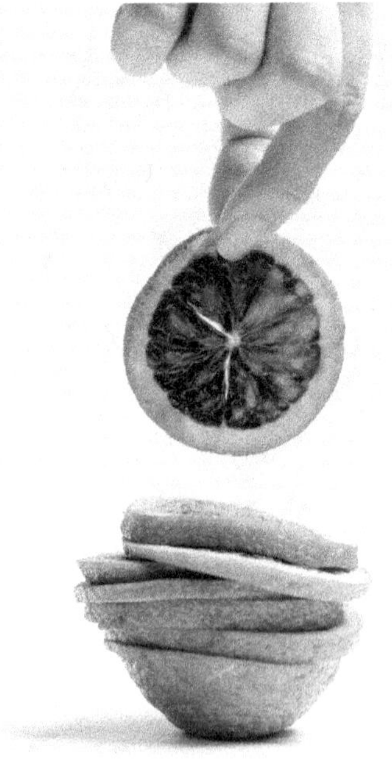

unusual cuisines that have made their way to Galveston's dining tables.

This chapter is a celebration of the island's ethnic richness and the confluence of different cuisines that mark Galveston's culinary scene.

❖ **Coastal Fusion:** International Seafood

This section digs into the realm of Coastal Fusion, a delightful combination of Galveston's seafood riches and cosmopolitan influences. Consider meals that mix Gulf shrimp with Asian flavors, or Gulf snapper with a Mediterranean flare.

You'll learn how to mix foreign tastes with local seafood, resulting in meals that actually represent Galveston's worldwide culinary variety.

❖ **Tex-Mex by the Sea:** Mexican-Texan Fusion

Galveston's closeness to Mexico has affected its Tex-Mex cuisine, and this part shows the art of mixing Mexican and Texan tastes.

Learn how to prepare Gulf shrimp tacos with a splash of spice or Tex-Mex enchiladas packed with seafood.

You'll discover how to bring a beach flavor to Tex-Mex cuisine.

❖ **Continental Classics:** European Elegance

European food has made its stamp on Galveston's culinary scene, and in this area, you'll appreciate the elegance of Continental classics.

Consider meals like French-inspired seafood bouillabaisse or Italian spaghetti with Gulf tastes. Learn how to lend European flare to Galveston's seafood delicacies.

Asian Delights from the Pacific Rim

The colorful tastes of the Pacific Rim make their way into Galveston's cuisine, and this section takes you on a tour through Asian influences.

Consider Thai-style Gulf snapper or Japanese sushi with a Gulf Coast flavor. You'll learn how to cook Asian-inspired seafood meals that mix tradition and originality.

Caribbean and Beyond Island-Inspired Global Fare

Galveston's tropical setting attracts Caribbean and worldwide influences, resulting in a unique blend of tastes. This area offers recipes that merge Caribbean flavors with Gulf seafood, as well as island-inspired cocktails that take you to tropical paradises.

Learn how to cook cosmopolitan cuisine with an island twist Chapter 8 is a worldwide feast that honors the different cuisines available in Galveston's culinary scene.

By the conclusion of this chapter, you'll not only know how to create a variety of strange and wonderful cuisine, but you'll also have a better sense of the island's cultural depth and ability to integrate foreign tastes into a tapestry of experiences.

Each dish represents the essence of international fusion, encouraging you to enjoy the world's gastronomic variety right in the heart of Galveston.

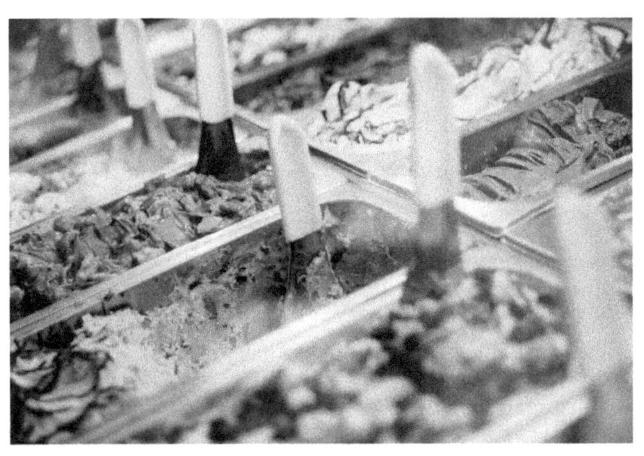

Asian Fusion Seafood Stir-Fry

Prepare to embark on an amazing culinary voyage in Chapter 8 of "The Galveston Cookbook" as we explore the area of Asian Fusion Seafood Stir-Fry.

This recipe is a magnificent mix of Galveston's coastal richness with the vivid tastes of Asia, culminating in a symphony of flavors and textures.

- ❖ **A Culinary Fusion**: Seafood from Galveston Meets Asian Flair

  Consider a hot wok loaded with Gulf shrimp, juicy crab, and delicate snapper, all dancing in a fragrant, savory sauce.

  The Asian Fusion Seafood Stir-Fry pays respect to the gastronomic fusion that distinguishes Galveston's eclectic palette.

  This part will show you how to blend Gulf seafood with the rich and exotic fragrances of Asia.

- ❖ **A Gulf Coast Tradition:** Choosing the Freshest Catch

The choice of the freshest seafood is at the center of this feast. Discover the value of choosing huge Gulf shrimp, sweet crab, and flaky snapper to produce a stir-fry rich in marine flavor.

Recognize the relationship between ethical seafood purchases and the preservation of the Gulf's natural resources.

❖ **Asian Flavors:** Infusing Seafood in Galveston

The sauce and spices are the key to a wonderful Asian Fusion Seafood Stir-Fry. In this lesson, you'll learn how to produce a tasty sauce using soy, ginger, garlic, and other aromatic components.

Learn how to produce the precise combination of sweet, savory, and umami tastes that distinguish Asian food.

The Precision and Speed of Stir-Frying

Stir-frying is a talent that demands both accuracy and rapidity.

In this part, you'll master the principles of high-heat cooking, ensuring that your seafood stays soft and tasty.

Recognize the necessity of constant movement and speedy cooking to develop a meal brimming with brilliant colors and textures.

❖ **Garnishing and Presentation:** A Senses Feast

Garnishing and presentation are the finishing touches to your Asian Fusion Seafood Stir-Fry. Consider a bright variety of fresh herbs, lively veggies, and aromatic sesame seeds gracing your dish.

Learn how to make a visually pleasing and delectable presentation that is a feast for both the eyes and the palate.

❖ **Savoring the Stir-Fry:** A Culinary Harmony

Asian Fusion Seafood Stir-Fry is more than simply a dinner; it's a culinary symphony in which the tastes of Galveston's seafood merge with the fragrant essence of Asia.

By the conclusion of this segment, you'll not only have a fantastic supper but also a deeper knowledge of the island's various culinary influences.

Each mouthful reflects the spirit of fusion, inviting you to experience the exquisite blend of Galveston's coastal richness with the vibrant and bold tastes of Asia—a supper that is not only a treat for the taste buds but also a culinary voyage of discovery.

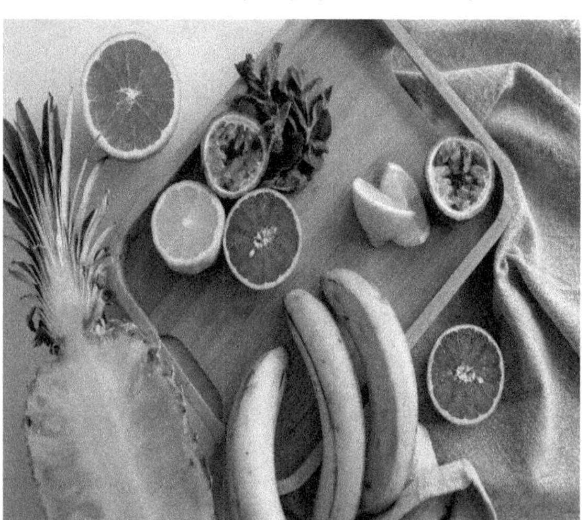

Mediterranean-Inspired Stuffed Bell Peppers

In Chapter 8 of "The Galveston Cookbook," we travel on a Mediterranean-inspired culinary trip with "Mediterranean-Inspired Stuffed Bell Peppers.

" These bell peppers mix the coastal elements of Galveston with the rich, sweet tastes of the Mediterranean.

A Mediterranean Odyssey: The Coastal Bounty of Galveston Meets the Mediterranean

Consider colorful bell peppers filled to the brim with a wonderful blend of Gulf shrimp, fresh herbs, rice, and fragrant spices. Mediterranean-Inspired.

The stuffed bell peppers witness to the gourmet combination that happens when Galveston's beachside luxury meets the richness of Mediterranean cuisine.

In this chapter, you'll uncover the key to producing this substantial and flavorful dinner.

Choosing the Most Fresh Ingredients: Gulf Coast Freshness

The selection of components is vital to this cuisine. Learn how to pick the freshest bell peppers, Gulf shrimp, and herbs to ensure that every mouthful explodes with bright flavors. Recognize the relationship between obtaining local foods and maintaining the authenticity of Galveston's coastal gems.

Creating the Filling with Mediterranean Flavors

It takes an artisan to produce the right Mediterranean-inspired filling. In this episode, you'll discover how to blend Gulf shrimp, aromatic rice, garlic, herbs like oregano and basil, and a splash of olive oil to create a Mediterranean-inspired concoction. Learn how to create a balanced combination of textures and fragrances.

- ❖ **The Stuffing Art:** Precision and Care
  Stuffed bell peppers demand accuracy and attention in their preparation. Learn how to hollow out the peppers and load them with the Mediterranean-inspired filling.

Understand the requirement of meticulous packing to ensure that each pepper is packaged precisely.

❖ **Baking and Presentation:** A Senses Feast

Baking and presentation are the finishing touches to your Mediterranean-inspired Stuffed Bell Peppers.

Imagine the peppers rising from the oven, their vivid colors and pungent fragrances filling the kitchen. Learn how to gain the optimal baking time for delicate, tasty peppers.

Discover the garnishing and presentation strategy that converts your cuisine into a sensory feast.

Savoring the Stuffed Peppers at a Mediterranean Feast Mediterranean-Inspired Stuffed Bell Peppers are a Mediterranean feast in which Galveston's maritime characteristics are taken to new heights with fragrant Mediterranean spices and herbs.

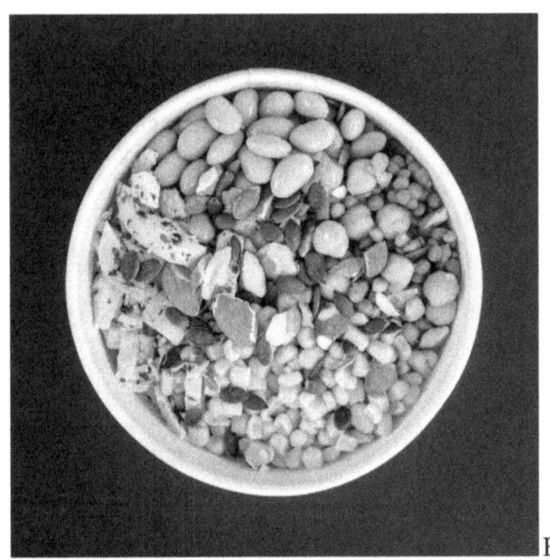By the conclusion of this portion, you'll have not only a fantastic lunch but also a deeper awareness of the island's potential to embrace different culinary influences.

Each mouthful reflects the spirit of fusion, encouraging you to experience the exquisite blend of Galveston's coastal richness with the rich and fragrant fragrances of the Mediterranean—a dinner that is not only a feast for the taste buds but a Mediterranean adventure　　　on　　　a　　　plate.

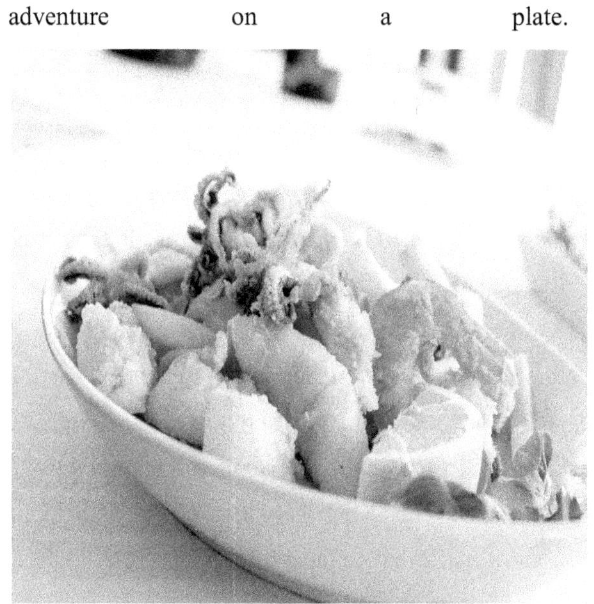

Galveston's Global Spice Market

Enter the intriguing world of Chapter 8 of "The Galveston Cookbook" as we study "Galveston's Global Spice Market." This part is a delectable voyage across the globe, exhibiting the rich tapestry of spices that have made their way into the island's cuisine.

Aromatic Avenues: Spice Traditions in Galveston

Imagine yourself wandering through the busy aisles of Galveston's spice market, surrounded by a kaleidoscope of colors and a symphony of fragrances.

Galveston's Global Spice Market serves as a tribute to the island's particular culinary traditions and enthusiasm for combining spices from all across the globe.

In this part, you'll learn about the power of spices and how they can turn ordinary dishes into extraordinary gourmet experiences.

❖ **Spice Selection:** A Flavorful World

The selection of spices is at the center of this gourmet trip.

Discover the vast selection of spices available in Galveston, from the heat of Indian curry powders to the smokiness of Mexican chipotle peppers and the pungency of Middle Eastern za'atar.

Recognize how each spice has a particular personality and may improve your cuisine in a number of ways.

❖ **The Blending Art:** Spice Mixtures & Seasonings

Developing spice mixes and spices is an art form that adds depth and complexity to your cuisine. In this part, you'll learn how to blend spices to produce distinct flavors and rubs. Learn how to balance tastes, produce the perfect degree of heat, and design spice mixes customized to Galveston's cuisine.

Culinary Creations with Spices

Spices are the hidden heroes who turn everyday cuisine into magnificent culinary creations. In this segment, you'll look at a range of foods that illustrate the adaptability of spices. From fragrant curries to spicy rubs for Gulf shrimp, you'll discover how to embellish your recipes with exotic tastes.

- ❖ **Keeping Spices Fresh:** Storage and Care

  Spices must be preserved and maintained correctly to keep their strength and taste. In this part, you'll learn about the best methods to store spices, from selecting the correct containers to knowing shelf life.

  Learn how to keep your spice collection fresh and flavorful.

- ❖ **A World of Flavor:** Savoring the Spice Traditions of Galveston

  The Global Spice Market in Galveston is more than just ingredients; it's a cultural experience that links you to the world's culinary history. By the conclusion of this session, you'll not only have a selection of scrumptious dishes under your belt but also a broader awareness   of   the

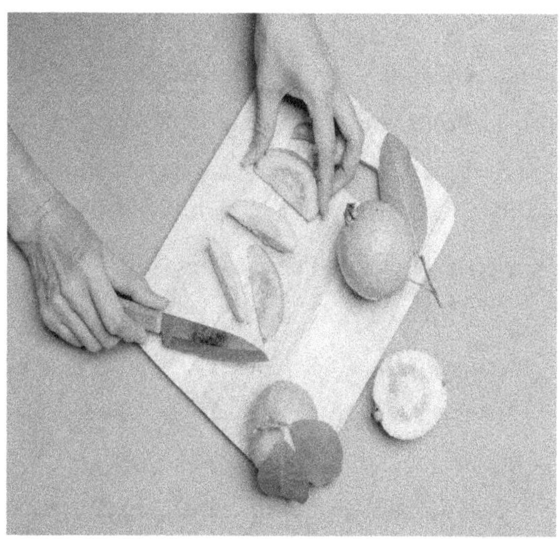

island's love of exotic spices.

Each dish captures the essence of spice, encouraging you to sample the rich tapestry of tastes that define Galveston's worldwide culinary traditions—a trip that is more than just about cuisine, but also a celebration of the world's spice bazaar right at your fingertips.

| GALVESTON COOKBOOK RECIPE

are preserved in jars of joy. Consider jars of pickled shrimp, peppery relishes, and homemade jams. You'll learn how to preserve seasonal products, enabling you to enjoy Galveston's delicacies all year.

- ❖ **Heirlooms and Family Recipes**

  The lifeblood of Galveston's culinary culture is family recipes. This section dives into the necessity of handing down beloved recipes and artifacts from generation to generation.

  Learn about the history of Galveston families and their links to the island's culture through these dishes.

- ❖ **Historical Re-Creation**: Food Traditions in Galveston

  Typically, sustaining Galveston's culinary legacy includes re-creating previous feasts that have been cherished for decades. This section will take you back in time to uncover iconic dinners that have marked the island's gastronomic traditions.

  Learn to appreciate history through your culinary creations.

- ❖ **Culinary Documentation and Storytelling**

  Culinary history is more than simply recipes; it's also about storytelling. In this part, we analyze the significance of maintaining family tales, recipes, and oral traditions that preserve the spirit of Galveston's culinary culture. Learn how to preserve the memories and anecdotes related with your favorite dish.

- ❖ **The Community's Role: Culinary Celebrations**

  Community gatherings and culinary events play a crucial part in sustaining Galveston's culinary culture. In this part, you'll learn the power of gathering together to share food, stories, and customs.

  Learn how these events promote community relationships and preserve the continuation of Galveston's culinary culture.

  Chapter 9 is a great monument to the island's commitment to maintain its culinary traditions. By the conclusion of this chapter, you'll not only have a collection of time-honored recipes, but also a deeper knowledge of the island's regard for tradition and the necessity of passing on the tastes that characterize Galveston's culture.

Each meal reflects the essence of Galveston's culinary legacy, pushing you to relish the joys of the past while looking forward—a celebration of the island's ancient food traditions and the people who keep them alive.

Traditional Galveston Pickling Techniques

Enter the delightful world of Chapter 10.1 of "The Galveston Cookbook" as we unveil the mysteries of "Traditional Galveston Pickling Techniques.

" This section commemorates Galveston's time-honored traditions of preserving the island's bright vegetables and seafood by pickling.

- ❖ **A Look Back in Time:** Galveston's Pickling Tradition

  Consider a bright kitchen with glass jars sparkling on wooden shelves and overflowing with a variety of pickled delights.

  Traditional Galveston Pickling Techniques bring you back in time, and keeping the tastes of the island was a labor of love. In this session, you'll discover the age-old practice of pickling, a process that assures Galveston's harvest may be enjoyed all year.

❖ **The Pickling Ingredients:** The Essence of Preservation

The selection of components is vital to pickling. Discover how to select the finest Gulf shrimp, crisp cucumbers, and fragrant herbs and spices for pickled delicacies.

Discover how the mix of fresh vegetables and fragrant spices gives the essence of preservation.

How to Make Pickling Liquids with Brine and Vinegar

Making the right brine or vinegar solution is important to pickling success. This section will show you how to produce tasty pickling liquids that will infuse your vegetables with a spicy punch.

Learn how to balance sweetness, acidity, and spices to obtain the right taste profile.

❖ **The Packing Art:** Preparing Jars and Ingredients

Pickling comes to life during the hard process of packing jars. Consider cucumbers snuggled amid dill sprigs, or Gulf shrimp piled high with onions and spices.

Learn how to clean, sanitize, and fill jars with components to guarantee a safe and fun pickling procedure.

❖ **Timing and Patience:** Pickling Time

Traditional pickling demands a lot of patience. In this part, you'll grasp the necessity of letting your pickled creations to rest and develop their tastes over time.

Learn about the appropriate pickling periods for various components and how patience pays off with the highest effects.

❖ **Savoring Pickled Treasures:** Culinary Pleasure

Traditional Galveston Pickling Techniques give more than simply preserved food; they also convey a flavor of history and heritage.

By the conclusion of this segment, you'll not only have a cherished collection of pickling recipes, but also a stronger connection to the island's culinary heritage.

Each jar captures the spirit of Galveston's pickling heritage, encouraging you to appreciate the flavors of preservation and time-honored techniques—an appetizing journey that is more than just about taste, but also a celebration of Galveston's rich culinary history and the love that goes into every pickled treasure.

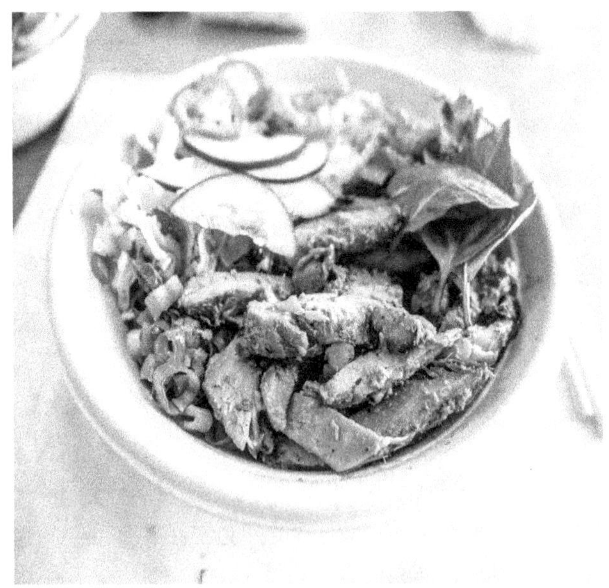

Home Canning and Jam Making

Enter the cozy world of "The Galveston Cookbook" Chapter 9 as we study the great talent of "Home Canning and Jam Making." This part is a lovely excursion into Galveston's heritage of conserving seasonal treasures and making tasty jams that symbolize the island's culture.

- ❖ **Timeless Preservation:** Galveston's Home Canning Heritage

  Consider a bright kitchen filled with the tantalizing scent of cooked fruit and the subtle clinking of glass jars. Home Canning and Jam Making are culinary traditions that bridge the gap between the present and the past.

  In this part, you'll learn how to preserve Galveston's seasonal abundance and prepare tasty, aromatic jams.

The selection of components is vital to home canning and jam manufacturing. Learn how to gather the ripest berries, juiciest peaches, and best figs that Galveston's land has to offer. Recognize how the quality of your ingredients affects the final flavor of your jams and canned meals.

❖ **Jam Making Magic:** Making Sweet Spreads

Jam making is an art form in which fruit is converted into delectable spreads. In this part, you'll learn how to produce vivid, delectable jams by boiling fruits with sugar and possibly a touch of citrus.

Discover how to acquire the perfect set, balance sweetness, and produce jams that pop with the flavor of Galveston's abundance.

❖ **The Canning Art:** Preserving Goodness

Canning is the cornerstone of food preservation. This section will show you how to can jams and other delicacies step by step. From sterilizing jars to correctly sealing them, you'll learn how to keep your preserved delights fresh and secure.

Labeling and Storing Jars of Memories

It is crucial to label and preserve your canned goods and jams to retain their quality. This section will educate you about labeling techniques that reflect the spirit of Galveston's culinary culture. Learn how to keep your creations so that they may be enjoyed for months, if not years, to come.

❖ **Traditional Flavors:** Homemade Jams and Canned Goods

Home Canning and jam-making are more than simply culinary activities; they convey a feeling of tradition and commitment.

By the conclusion of this segment, you'll not only have a cherished collection of recipes but also a better grasp of the island's devotion to maintaining its seasonal resources.

Each jar and spoonful captures the essence of Galveston's homey, nurturing culinary heritage, inviting you to savor the flavors of tradition and the warmth.

That goes into every homemade jam and preserved good—an edible journey that is more than just about taste, but also a celebration of Galveston's rich culinary history and the love that goes into every jar.

Recipes Passed Down Through Generations

In Chapter 9 of "The Galveston Cookbook," we celebrate "Recipes Passed Down Through Generations." This section takes you deep into the hearts of Galveston's families and the beloved recipes that have been carefully shared down the years.

The Taste of Tradition: Family Recipes from Galveston

Consider an ancient, ripped recipe card, replete with scribbled notes and family secrets.

Recipes Passed Down Through Generations

---

encapsulate the spirit of Galveston's culinary culture, where meals function as time capsules, preserving memories and establishing relationships. In this segment, you'll learn about the persistent effect of family recipes.

- ❖ **Generational Connection:** From Grandmother to Grandchild

  Family recipes are the connections that bind generations. In this part, we look at the joy of passing recipes down from grandmother to grandson, mother to daughter, and father to son.

  Discover how these culinary traditions become engrained in the family's identity and history.

- ❖ **Success Secrets: Mastering Traditional Dishes**

  Traditional foods often show wisdom obtained through experience. This section digs into the methods and secrets that enable outstanding recipes to endure the test of time.

  Learn how to tackle the intricacies of traditional Galveston recipes and make culinary wonders that bring nostalgia and delight.

- ❖ **A History Celebration:** Re-creating Family Classics

  Recipes passed down through generations are more than simply instructions; they are tales waiting to be shared. This part will show you how to reproduce family classics that recount the history of Galveston's family.

Learn how to respect the past while putting your own touch on family favorites.

- ❖ **Culinary Heirlooms:** Preserving and Sharing Memories

Family recipes are culinary gold mines. This section will look at the necessity of sharing and preserving these life-changing occurrences. Understand how documenting and sharing family recipes ensures that they will be handed down for decades to come, carrying the torch of Galveston's culinary history.

- ❖ **Savoring Family Traditions: A Taste of Love**

Recipes that have been handed down through generations are more than simply about food; they also contain a flavor of love, history, and shared experiences.

By the conclusion of this part, you'll not only have a collection of cherished recipes but also a better awareness of the island's reverence for tradition and the necessity of passing on the tastes that characterize.

Galveston's culture each dish captures the essence of Galveston's culinary heritage, inviting you to savor the flavors of tradition, love, and the enduring connections.

that family recipes bring—an edible journey that is more than just about taste but a heartfelt celebration of Galveston's rich culinary history and the bonds that bind generations together.

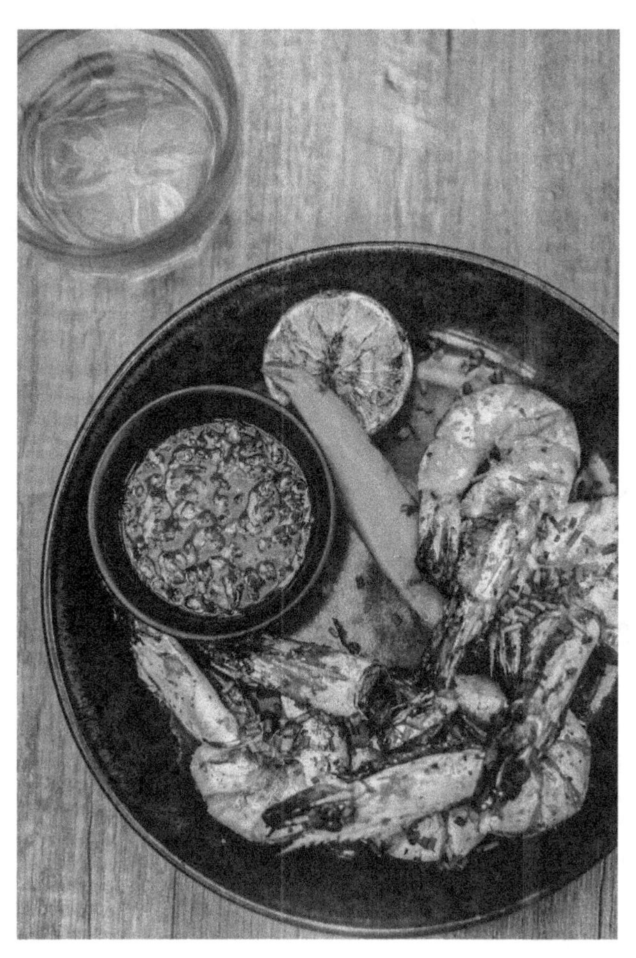

GALVESTON COOKBOOK RECIPE

Conclusion

We've been on a gastronomic trip with "The Galveston Cookbook," learning about the flavors, cultures, and tales that define the food on this bustling island. From the fresh Gulf seafood to the worldwide influences that have influenced its cuisine, each chapter has been a celebration of Galveston's rich culinary past.

We've discovered ways to preserve Galveston's seasonal plenty, creating jams, pickles, and recipes that encapsulate the essence of the island's prosperity. We've enjoyed seafood delicacies and relished in the warmth of family traditions passed down through generations.

"The Galveston Cookbook" is a love letter to the island's culture, a tribute to the individuals who bring the island's culinary traditions to life, and a reminder of the enduring link between food and the heart. It displays Galveston's capacity to merge the ancient and the new, the local and the world, in a tapestry of flavors that genuinely engage the senses.

As we end our culinary adventure, may you leave with not just the recipes but also a better understanding of Galveston's soul, a connection to its past, and an appreciation for the passion and care that goes into each meal. "The Galveston Cookbook" allows you to explore not only the flavors, but also the tales, traditions, and memories that make Galveston cuisine a true culinary treasure. Roll up your sleeves, gather your ingredients, and let the spirit of the island guide you as you go on your own culinary journey inspired by Galveston's rich culinary legacy.

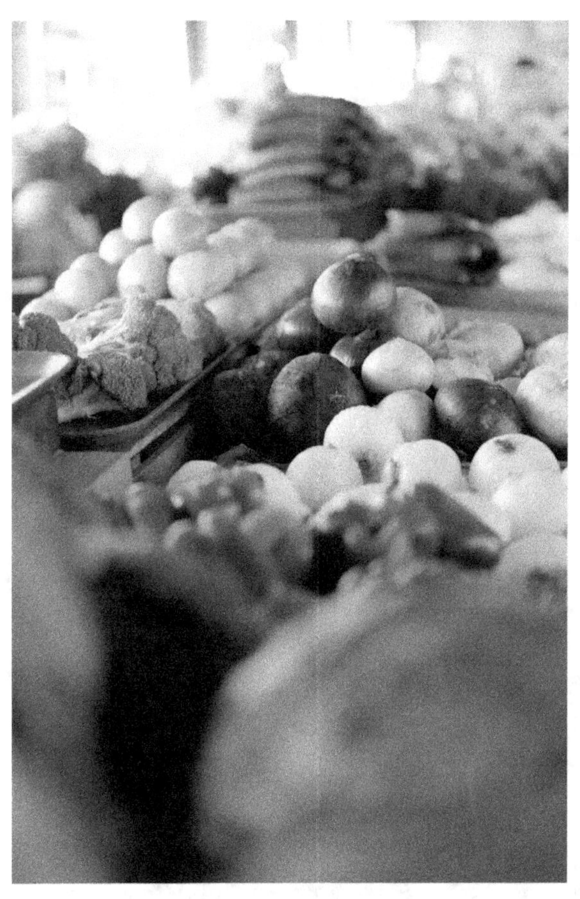

| GALVESTON COOKBOOK RECIPE

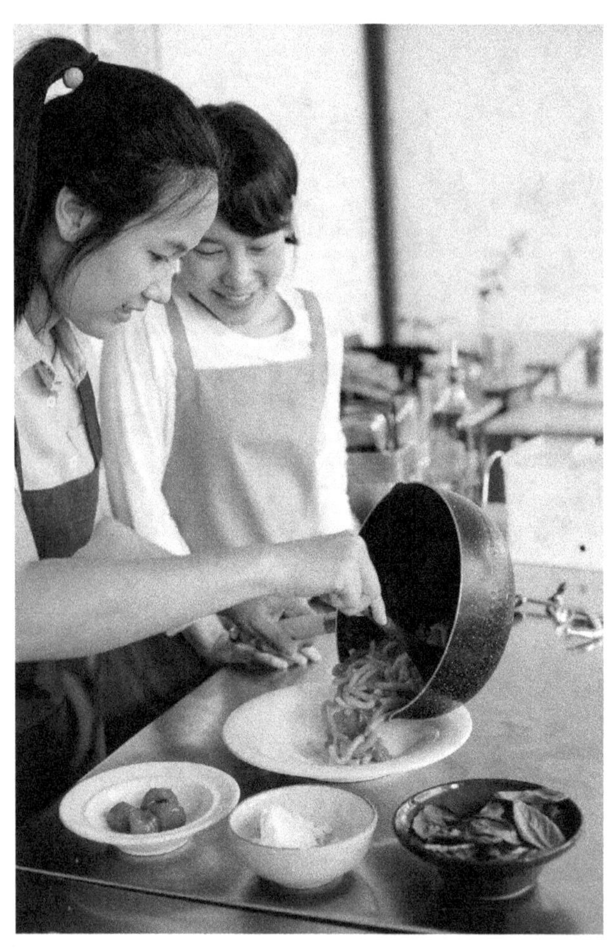

GALVESTON COOKBOOK RECIPE